healthy solutions

A Guide to Simple Healing and Healthy Wisdom

David N. Russell, Ph.D., M.F.A.
with Lynn Wiese Sneyd

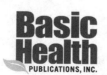

Basic Health
PUBLICATIONS, INC.

The information contained in this book is based upon the research and personal and professional experiences of the authors. It is not intended as a substitute for consulting with your physician or other healthcare provider. Any attempt to diagnose and treat an illness should be done under the direction of a healthcare professional.

The publisher does not advocate the use of any particular healthcare protocol but believes the information in this book should be available to the public. The publisher and authors are not responsible for any adverse effects or consequences resulting from the use of the suggestions, preparations, or procedures discussed in this book. Should the reader have any questions concerning the appropriateness of any procedures or preparation mentioned, the authors and the publisher strongly suggest consulting a professional healthcare advisor.

Basic Health Publications, Inc.
28812 Top of the World Drive
Laguna Beach, CA 92651
949-715-7327

Library of Congress Cataloging-in-Publication Data

Russell, David
    Healthy solutions : a guide to simple healing and healthy wisdom /
David Russell, with Lynn Wiese Sneyd.
        p. cm.
    Includes bibliographical references and index.
    ISBN-13: 978-1-59120-108-3 (alk. paper)
    ISBN-10: 1-59120-108-X
    1. Medicine, Popular. 2. Health. 3. Self-care, Health. I. Sneyd, Lynn
Wiese. II. Title.

    RC81.R96   2006
    616—dc22

                                                            2006003329

Editor: John Anderson
Copyeditor: Susan Andrews
Typesetting/Book design: Gary A. Rosenberg
Cover design: Mike Stromberg

Printed in the United States of America

10 9 8 7 6 5 4 3 2 1

Contents

PART THREE *The Therapeutic Nature of Foods*

To the love that has made this book possible:
my wife, Tine,
my children, Nathan, Mark, Miriam, Rebecca, and Bine,
my parents,
my sister,
my patients,
and the compassionate and beautiful minds
from whom I have had the privilege of learning.

May this book serve the innocence of the heart.

"And all things, and all manner of things will be well."
(Julian of Norwich)

—David Russell

※ ※ ※

For my children and future generations.
May you embrace these concepts with reverence and awe.

—Lynn Wiese Sneyd

Acknowledgments

A special thanks to Sheree Bykofsky and Janet Rosen for nestling this book in a home and to our publisher Norman Goldfind, our editor John Anderson, and the staff at Basic Health Publications for making the home welcoming and comfortable.

Foreword

Healthy Solutions constitutes a radically refreshing way to approach healing. My first response upon reading this book was pure joy coupled with the wondrous feeling that caring for the body is a great adventure. In fact, I felt healthier just from reading and thinking about this masterful work. I suspect that you will feel something similar after digesting the following pages.

The book is rich with information and perspectives that nourish the body, mind, and spirit. These days, when we approach medical information, we often expect to respond with an element of fear. Not so here—the tone and contents of this book, while exuding expertise and knowledge, are filled with love and wisdom that instill a sense of confidence in our ability to care for our bodies and confidence that our bodies will respond to such self-care.

In our age, a false flight from the pain of every sort of illness, nurtured by the strictly modern fantasy that a technical approach to medicine can restore health, has effectively eliminated the concept that illness plays an important role in our growth and maturation. Illness is taken to be the opposite of health, and the more aggressively it is fought against, the better. However, health and illness are polarities of relationship in our ever-growing experience of life, rather than opposites in a struggle. We are always living somewhere between these polarities. Only when there is radical imbalance do we typically need the assistance of medical intervention.

The illnesses described in this book can be effectively worked with by remembering that there can be health only when there is also illness. We are seldom one without the other, even when we feel more or less well. In fact, the notion that there can be health without illness leads to a decidedly unhealthy and unintegrated way of perceiving life. The brilliant psychologist Carl Jung defined neurosis as one-sidedness, and by that he meant we are out of balance when we have excessive singularity of orientation.

This book helps us gain new insight into health and illness. We are invited to see that a headache might have to do with the digestion, that the liver is connected with the eye, and that a symptom wants to lead us into a mystery story. Illness is often a signal to care for the body, listen to it as we would a captivating storyteller, rather than taking it in for repair. It is entirely possible that one can have absolutely no visible symptoms and actually be very ill and that medications can cover our suffering while failing to touch the source of our illness. The worst misery is not to be aware of misery, to have lost all imagination of suffering other than the overriding thought that it must be excised as quickly as possible.

While reading this work, one can't help but feel the wholeness of David and Lynn's approach. It is a work of wisdom. Wisdom is a way of knowing and works differently from ordinary intelligence: it works with polarities without splitting them apart; it is a way of knowing something from within, by communion and intimacy, rather than by being a spectator and theorizing. Wisdom contemplates more than analyzes; it adds empathy to insight. You can't help but feel centuries of wise practice speak through this writing, bringing confidence, comfort, and reverence to health and illness.

One of the truly valuable contributions of this writing is the way in which the wisdom of Classical medicine—which includes traditional practices such as Chinese medicine and acupuncture, Western herbal medicine, homeopathy, Tibetan medicine, and Ayurvedic medicine, to name a few—is applied in ways appropriate to our present lives and circumstances. This book distills the essence of these healing traditions and shows their many applications in more fully understanding the body and in developing helpful, yet simple remedies.

You will, through reading this book, be empowered to take responsibility for your own healing. The results of prescription drugs are often immediate and dramatic because only the symptoms are addressed. Preparing and working with these remedies may or may not produce those kinds of dramatic results, because the underlying system that is ill is being addressed rather than the symptoms. But when you take responsibility for your health and healing, you enter into a process in which your conscious engagement is a vital part of the process.

To begin to question some of the tenants of modern mechanistic medicine and turn toward other approaches not only takes time, it takes new learning. Perhaps the most wonderful aspect of this book is that the authors provide us with a very careful and full understanding of the human body, an approach that utilizes the concepts of modern physiology, but sees them in a more holistic context. You will begin to experience the incredible, mysterious wisdom of the body. Everything that happens within our bodily organism is for the health of the body, even those processes that seem to signify illness. In fact, those symptoms always signify the body engaging in the healing process. Once this simple yet exquisitely profound concept is truly under-stood and experienced, you are on the way to practicing the art of healing.

—Robert Sardello, Ph.D., Director, The School of Spiritual Psychology, and author of *Freeing the Soul from Fear* and *The Power of Soul*

Introduction

This book was written for you. Before explaining how to use it, I'd like to explain how it came into being. I have been working in the field of medicine for more than thirty years, mostly in the general clinical practices of natural medicine and integrated medicine, primarily in Europe and more recently in the United States.

Ten years ago, I met Lynn Wiese Sneyd and her family, who consulted me as a doctor. Traditionally, part of a doctor's responsibility is to educate patients. Throughout my career, I have been interested in this educational process and have conducted lectures and seminars on many aspects of health and healing in order to assist individuals in taking control of their health. Shortly after meeting Lynn, I organized a seminar called "Self-Healing in Ayurvedic and Tibetan Medicines" to be held in Khatmandu, Nepal. Lynn's interest in natural, holistic philosophies of health had been increasing steadily. As a young mother, she wanted to understand and respond to her family's health issues, rather than rely exclusively on an HMO or private doctor and the inevitable prescription drugs. Lynn and her husband decided to journey to the other side of the world to attend the seminar.

Lynn's journey to Nepal, coupled with the ensuing lifestyle changes she gradually introduced at home, formed themselves into an excellent book called *Holistic Parenting: Raising Children to a New Physical, Emotional, and Spiritual Well-Being* (Los Angeles: Keats Publishing, 2000), a sympathetic and informative recounting of her exasperations, doubts, and discoveries. I was privileged to be able to help Lynn with the medical aspects of her book. From our work together, the concept of a new book formed.

When we first thought of doing this book, the plan was to compile some short notes for family and friends. The concept, however, quickly expanded into a comprehensive, how-to book that recommends simple home remedies and treatments that are safe and effective, having proven themselves in the clinical practices of natural medicine. In addition, informative health sections clarify and educate about the nature of health and disease and describe the processes and functions of the body. We feel that understanding the body is as important as finding the appropriate way of treating it.

The book consists of three parts. The first part provides information on general health topics that you can read at your leisure and that will help you understand the ways natural medicine views health, disease, and healing. What does the body mean when it uses the language of symptoms? How and why does the body function as an integrated system? How does the immune system function as a system of integration and not merely a defense mechanism within the body? How does standard medical practice differ from natural medical practice? What is meant by *Classical medicine,* a term that we use throughout the book? The information presented in each chapter has been gathered from the many traditions within the realm of natural health and healing.

The second part addresses specific ailments, providing clear and simple information about how to treat the uncomplicated acute symptoms that we all experience at one time or another in our lives. These symptoms include sore throats, earaches, coughs, headaches, and digestive problems. Each chapter is devoted to one subject and is divided into two sections. Section one is called a "teaching." In the practice of Classical medicine, the doctor is considered a learned teacher as well as a skilled therapist. It is as much the doctor's responsibility to inform and educate his or her patients as it is to give medical treatments. This practice stems from the fact that Classical medicine considers ignorance of the laws of nature and appropriate lifestyle as being the major cause of illness. In each teaching section, you will learn about the specific functions of the body and mind from the perspective of Classical medicine and how to interpret the body's reactions when dealing with health issues. You will come to understand more about the marvelous and wise way the body and mind work. This knowledge will increase your confidence in supporting the healing process using simple and effective natural therapies that you can apply in the comfort and security of your home.

Section two of each chapter focuses on actual therapies. The information presented is easy to follow and does not require you to have any previous knowledge of medicine or of treating disease. We recommend therapies that you are likely to have on hand or can easily obtain at any grocery store. We have avoided recommending treatments that are too complicated to be used without prior medical knowledge or remedies that are only available at specialty stores.

The third part of the book deals with the therapeutic nature of foods. It includes a chapter called Materia Medica, which describes the therapeutic effects of foods and remedies and how to use them. This information has been gathered from the best sources of natural health practice in Europe and the Classical medical sciences from Ayurvedic, Chinese, Tibetan, and Islamic traditions. These perspectives and methods have proven themselves effective through the last six centuries and, in some cases, even longer.

Although the natural healing methods outlined in this book are very effective, they cannot deal with all situations. Emergencies or life-threatening problems as well as recurring health issues require the help of a specialist. When in doubt, contact a competent natural healthcare professional or doctor.

HEALTH AND HEALING

You must never forget that when working with your health, either to support and maintain it or to resolve a specific health issue, you are dealing with the most complex living organism on the planet. You are a marvelous unity of body, emotions, mind, and spirit, all working together in a single person. Health, by definition, deals with the *whole* person because health belongs to the whole person and does not consist solely of the body and its tissues or the mind and its emotions. Your life and health are dependent on the simultaneous and integrated functioning of all your biological systems, as well as on the domain of your mind and spirit.

Because health is something that belongs to you, your health is *your* issue, not the doctor's or therapist's. Health is very intimate and personal, and only you can take the responsibility for what to do and how it should be done. When we have a health issue, we usually consult a doctor and leave everything up to him or her. We don't always question or attempt to understand the whats and whys of how we got into the situation or how a treatment will affect us. Essentially, we cut ourselves off from being present and interactive in the most intimate and important aspect of our lives—our personal health.

We have slipped into this habit because we see ourselves primarily as clinical objects, reduced to our chemical processes and tissues. Though the clinical viewpoint is an important parameter in an overall perspective of health, other essential points must be included. Health and healing are first and foremost matters of care and compassion. To heal, we need to feel cared for and intimately involved with our healing process, as well as have a sense that others, including the doctor, truly care for us and desire to help us. We need to understand that though the symptoms of a particular health issue might manifest only in the body, they affect our entire person—body, mind, and spirit—and that we need to access the healing mechanisms of our whole being. Healing is not just a matter of eliminating a symptom but deeply involves our process of growth and development as a person. We can only heal when we are willing to become truly active and present in our own healing processes. Doctors and therapists can't make us healthy; they can only support the will of the body, mind, and spirit and its innate healing ability to help us become whole and healthy.

This book invites you to partake in this process of becoming whole and healthy. It provides a greater understanding of health, its issues, and the means by which you can become an active participant in this essential and beautiful part of life.

PART ONE

The Nature
of Health

CHAPTER 1

Cultural Perspectives of Medical Practice

In our culture, two predominant forms of medical practice serve our communities. One is the standard field of medicine with which we are all familiar, typically called "allopathic" or "conventional" medicine. Medical doctors, physician assistants, and nursing professionals, among others, practice this type of medicine. The other main form of health care involves the field of natural medicine, also called "Classical" or "holistic" medicine. Naturopaths, homeopaths, and acupuncturists, just to name a few, practice this type of medicine. Each of these systems has strengths and weaknesses. Each one can help us achieve our health goals and contribute positively to our quality of life. Although different in numerous ways, they remain complementary.

Conventional medical practice focuses on the presence of symptoms and disease. Its primary therapies involve chemical medicines (drugs), surgery, and so-called replacement therapy, in which the body is given substances, like hormones or other biochemical components, that for some reason it seems to lack. Often, a diagnosis involves tests that either quantify a substance in the body or show an image. Blood tests, x-rays, and magnetic resonance imagery (MRI) scans are among a multitude of diagnostic tests used to determine what is wrong with the body. Although some of these tests are highly sophisticated, they may not reveal the underlying *causes* of the problem.

All allopathic therapies, regardless of the type, have one thing in common: they force or manipulate the body to respond in a particular way. Chemical drugs influence the way the body is functioning and make it respond according to the power and nature of the chemicals in the medicine. A good example of this scenario is pain medication, which short-circuits the pain reflexes in the nerve system so that we don't feel the pain, even though the cause of the pain remains. When we force or manipulate the body's natural functions, however, we do not really heal it. Moreover, the side effects of chemical drugs frequently cause problems for biological systems other than the one being treated. Chemical medicine is most appropriate when we are facing serious acute problems that the body cannot resolve in any other way.

Another form of manipulation is surgery. As you may know, surgery is the removal or repair of a tissue or an organ that seems impaired. It can be very helpful and necessary in certain cases, when the tissues are damaged beyond the body's ability to repair them. Surgery helps many people who would otherwise be victims of accidents or incurable tissue problems in organs that have had serious problems and have not properly healed. Replacement therapy replaces something the body seems to lack. Rather than helping the body to produce on its own what it lacks, this approach replaces the missing or deficient substances. While it can help reduce symptoms initially, replacement therapy doesn't solve the causes of *why* the body is not functioning properly. In the long run, replacement therapy has a tendency to inhibit the body's natural processes.

Natural health practices differ from conventional medicine in a number of ways. First, they use a different approach to therapy and, second, they have a different way of understanding the processes and functions of the body. Their point of reference is health rather than disease. Natural therapies such as homeopathy, acupuncture, and herbal medicine have no true side effects when applied correctly because they do not overpower or manipulate the body's own functions as chemical medicines do. Instead, they provide the necessary support for the body so that it can reestablish its normal, healthy ways of functioning.

For example, let's say you have an earache. A conventional medical doctor probably would prescribe an antibiotic to kill the bacteria. A natural medical doctor would use therapies that support the immune system so that body can resolve the situation through its own healing mechanisms. The therapies, by their very nature, also work on the underlying causes that allowed the ear infection to develop in the first place.

These two apparently different medical traditions, conventional and natural medicine, are complementary. Each one is appropriate to use in specific situations because each has the ability to solve specific kinds of problems. In our society, the conventional medical establishment is beginning to recognize the important contributions of natural medicine. As a result, practitioners from different traditions of medicine are starting to collaborate for the benefit of the patient.

THE BODY AS MACHINE

The history of medicine spans centuries and covers vast areas of knowledge. To some extent, every culture has established its own medical sciences and traditions. We often forget, however, that all sciences are basically philosophies: they reveal the way people view and experience their world, as well as how they attempt to understand the nature of life. At any point in history, all of the sciences in any culture reflect the desires, goals, and hopes of its people.

When we study the history of medicine, we see that our Western medical science is based on a very different viewpoint from that of the medical sciences of other cultures. This difference does not mean our science is better or more advanced. Rather, it shows how we understand the concepts of health and disease and how these ideas mesh with the other goals and desires of our culture.

For the last four hundred years, the machine has dominated Western society. We desire high productivity, so we constantly strive to develop more effective technologies. We demand that these technologies and machines operate correctly and efficiently. Because our culture belongs to the Age of the Machine, we tend to view the universe as a complex machine and ourselves as mechanics fixing and repairing the faults, failings, and breakdowns of life.

Even nature is perceived as being composed of separate parts that we attempt to control in order to achieve our goals. The current trends in agriculture illustrate this point. The economic goal of higher crop production has led to the introduction of toxic chemicals, such as pesticides and fertilizers, into the earth and to the manipulation of genetic plant material—both of these methods alter nature. The negative consequences of these actions will probably never be fully known.

This mechanistic view extends into medicine. We are accustomed to thinking of our body, for instance, as a finely tuned machine that contains separate parts like the heart, stomach, bones, and muscles. We have sciences that describe and analyze these parts. Anatomy, for instance, identifies the parts of the body. Physiology differentiates between the various measurable chemical and physical reactions that occur in the parts of the body's anatomy. Pathology describes the measurable changes in the body's cells and tissues that create observable symptoms when the body is not functioning properly.

When a part of the body malfunctions, diagnostic tests that measure and quantify are often used. X-rays, for instance, show how organs and tissues look physically; an EMG measures nerve impulses; and blood tests analyze the types and amounts of chemicals and hormones found in the bloodstream.

Although these methods are helpful, they tend to limit our knowledge of the body and its functions to what instruments or machines can measure.

This perception of the body as a machine rather than a complex living organism also influences the types of treatments that conventional medicine develops. As discussed earlier, some treatments are foreign to the body's own systems and therefore force or manipulate the body to comply in a certain way in order to achieve a specific result. But even when that result is achieved, the body may not be restored to its natural state of health. Remember, only the body can cure itself. Healing is a natural function of the body and occurs when the body is able to use its innate healing mechanisms. Sometimes, of course, the body needs outside assistance during the healing process—surgery may be necessary or a chemical medicine may be the best way to help the body solve a serious acute situation. But whatever type of assistance is administered, it must support the body's natural healing processes and not interfere with them.

FIGHTING DISEASE VERSUS PROMOTING HEALTH

The body-as-machine philosophy has thwarted the practice of curing and preventing disease. Many view our modern conventional medicine as highly advanced and technical, but the extensive side effects of chemical medicines and surgical procedures often impair the basic health of the individual. For the last few centuries, conventional medical practice has focused on *fighting disease* rather than on *promoting health*. Our medical system has made great strides in surgery, for example, but has failed to understand the nature of basic health in the body. Conventional medicine defines health as being the absence of symptoms, a definition that in no way leads us to a concept of true health. It does not understand how to prevent disease from occurring or how to support a state of health in the body so that strong medicines, surgery, organ transplants, and genetic manipulation are *not* necessary.

In America, medical drug advertisements on television and in magazines inculcate the message that we need these drugs to become healthy and live a fulfilling life. We have become a nation of drug users and abusers. Statistics show that those over age fifty take an average of two prescription drugs per day in order to maintain their health. Even simple and natural immune processes like colds, the flu, and sore throats are often treated with strong antibiotics, all of which have side effects that compromise the healthy functioning of tissues and cells.

Chronic diseases like cancer, heart disease, and arthritis are so prevalent that we have come to accept them as normal conditions of life. Medical research is committed to designing more and more drugs, but fails to ask the obvious question: Why have we become so unhealthy? If we again turn to statistics, we see that serious chronic diseases have risen dramatically since the early 1950s. In this same fifty-year period, the amount and types of toxins we have been subjected to have also risen dramatically. We ingest more medicines and receive more vaccines than ever before. Our food is full of chemicals, and our water and air are loaded with toxic waste. We need to recognize the connection between our toxic way of life and the emergence of chronic diseases.

Toxins of all kinds challenge the human immune system. None of us go through life without experiencing the way in which our immune system helps us to develop and maintain our health. These "immune experiences" are the simple acute ailments we all have faced, including colds, simple flu, coughs, fevers, and ear infections. Issues like these are not really diseases as such, but responses from our healthy immune systems that help us rebalance when we're under lifestyle or environmental stress. These immune responses are the body's way of cleansing itself of toxins, which compromise its systems, and microbes that are no longer useful for the body's proper functioning. All of these responses show that we are not living in a world only for ourselves, but that we're sharing life with our whole environment and responding to its natural laws.

The inability to understand the nature of health is one of the great failures of conventional medicine. It explains why so many people are turning to holistic forms of diagnosis and treatment that are based on concepts of health, rather than waiting until disease processes are so advanced that they need invasive medical treatment. Slowly, we are aligning ourselves with medical traditions of cultures that have understood the fundamental role nature plays in the true mechanisms of health. From this perspective, nature is seen as an interrelated play of forces and events that directly affect not only the individual, but also the universe of which he or she is a part.

CHAPTER 2

Life and the Body

All forms in the universe, be they atoms, crystals, chemical compounds, or the tissues of the body, share two primary qualities:

- They are created by, and function by way of, life-forming energies shared in common with the whole universe.

- While using these energies to ensure their function, they simultaneously form new energy.

Everything that can be seen, weighed, and measured is the result of these two factors. The physical foundation of the body, and in fact the foundation of all organic life, including plants, animals, and microbes, is the cell. The same energies that create the stars, planets, and great nebulas of our universe are active within us creating our tissues and organs. These energies, which make up and sustain life, work in the cells of the body. The cell acts as a container for these universal energies so that they can perform in a focused way and provide a basis for our identity and for the necessary functions of the body and mind.

THE BODY'S CELLS

All cells are individual living organisms in their own right. In simple life forms like microbes, the organism is just a single cell, while in the more complex organisms, like humans and animals, the body is made up of billions of individual cells that make up tissue systems such as organs, bones, and muscles. Complex organisms like the human body require a steering system to integrate individual cells so that they always work together as a team, allowing the body to live and function as a whole and single unit. This steering is accomplished by two aspects of energy that continually create the functional patterns of the cells and their integration within the whole organism.

The first of these aspects is the constitution, a hereditary "biological template" that we receive at the moment of conception. It could also be called the "individual identity template" because it makes us the particular individual we are. It determines the basic ways in which we will function both physically and psychologically throughout our lives. Furthermore, it makes us unique individuals, different to some degree from all others physically and emotionally. This biological identity template is in turn nourished and guided by a more universal field of energy that works in the background of all individual forms and identities. It is built on the foundation of a universal consciousness that binds all of creation together in the unity of life.

In our usual view of the world, it is hard to imagine that all matter and energy contain "consciousness" and that this consciousness connects every event and every form, be it a chemical reaction, an atom, or a cell. For the last half century, the well-established sciences of quantum physics and fractal mathematics have shown that consciousness pervades the entire universe and connects everything within it. In quantum physics, this connection is called the "universal field" and means that the functions of our cells and their energies and chemistry are connected to everything else in the universe. All world religions refer to this connection and consciousness as a quality of the divine. In some ways, we're not as "separate" as we thought!

By looking at the basic structure of a cell, we can understand how it serves as the foundation of our life as well as how it connects us to the world of nature that surrounds us. All cells have a cell membrane that surrounds the living matter of the cell itself. This membrane not only encloses the cell material but also makes it possible for the cell to relate to everything outside of itself. Think of the cell membrane as a wall. We can say that a wall, whether it surrounds a castle, garden, or cell, creates a relationship of identity. A relationship can only exist between two individual identities; we cannot relate to anything that does not have a boundary, which makes it different and distinct from anything else. Membranes are nature's way of creating identity by enclosing universal processes within an individual form.

Cells serve as the shelter and home of life, much like the homes where we live and go to nourish ourselves, rest, and build ourselves up. They are the basic structures that support and nourish our identity. The very sense that we have about ourselves as being individual and unique persons begins in the cell with its surrounding cell membrane.

Just as we are composed of different organs, tissues, and biochemical processes, so a cell also contains organs and processes that make up its individual life. The cell has organs for reproduction, organs that digest and create energy through metabolic processes, and organs that contain RNA and DNA making the cell a complete living organism. In fact, one of the cell's organs, called the mitochondria, is a small primitive bacteria that at one time during evolution existed freely on the Earth's surface. Over vast amounts of time and the creation of more and more complex organisms, the mitochondria moved into the cell and became the mechanism that provides the body with its main biochemical energy. We might say that in each of our cells, we are carrying a little part of the life of the whole planet that surrounds us and sustains us.

A complex organism can only live because all the individual cells of its body cooperate and work together to sustain the diverse functions of the body and mind. Humans, being the most complex of all living organisms, create this cooperation not only through biophysical processes but also through the intimate pattern of personal identity. That's why our emotional and mental processes strongly affect the health of our cells. The development of our identity is called the individuation process; this process makes us aware of who we are in the deepest sense and controls the way in which our cells respond to our unique and personal way of living and being.

THE THREE EMBRYOLOGICAL TISSUE SYSTEMS

Conventional medicine has always been interested in the way the fetal child develops after conception. It is quite amazing to see how a few basic cells that emerge after conception and during pregnancy become a fully developed human being, replete with complex systems of cells, tissues, and organs. The scientific field specializing in the developments of the fetus is called embryology. Recent research in this area has shown that the embryological tissue systems formed within the first week of fetal life play a vital role in our physical and mental health. For this reason, we will spend a little time exploring the significance of the embryological tissue systems.

In the first week after conception, cells organize themselves into three distinct layers from which all our future tissues and organs develop. The first layer to develop is called the *endoderm* and forms the initial tissue system of the embryo. The tissues that evolve from the endoderm are concerned with our digestion and nutrition. Nature in its wisdom initiates the development of the endoderm cells first so that the fetal child can be nourished and begin to grow and develop. This process parallels the planting of a seed. The seed contains all of the codes and energies needed to produce the full plant, yet it also needs nutrients from the earth and water in order to unfold and grow. Human conception is like planting a seed containing the codes and energies of a full and unique human individual. The seed is planted in the "earth" of the mother's womb, which nourishes it throughout its development. Besides creating the digestive organs, the endoderm also develops the liver, pancreas, the inner surface of the lungs, and the thyroid gland.

Very shortly after the endoderm becomes active, the remaining two embryological tissue systems form and become activated. These are the *mesoderm* and *ectoderm*. The mesoderm develops the organs and tissues that eventually become the center balancing point of our minds and bodies and work to integrate the functions of the ectoderm and endoderm. The mesoderm tissues and organs include the heart, blood vessels, connective tissues, cartilage and bone tissue, muscles, blood, lymph, kidney, spleen, tooth pulp, and reproductive organs.

From the ectoderm comes the nerve tissues of our central, autonomic, and peripheral nerve systems that make up our brain, spinal cord, and the nerves that extend to our limbs and organs. In addition, the ectoderm develops our skin and its glands, hair, nails, and the outer enamel of our teeth.

EMBRYOLOGICAL TISSUE SYSTEMS AND HEALTH

In terms of our health, it is significant that the organs and tissues created in the embryological tissue system all remain functionally connected to one another throughout our life. This connection explains why the thyroid gland, for instance, is connected to metabolic processes in our digestive organs— both the digestive organs and the thyroid develop from the endoderm. When we assess symptoms, be they physical or mental, we need to evaluate the symptoms in terms of their relationship to the embryological tissue systems. In our example of the thyroid, Classical medicine usually resolves thyroid problems by working on the stomach organ because both were developed from the same embryological tissue and the Stomach Systems's energy channels control the thyroid's functions. This relationship, in turn, means that any chronic disturbances in the stomach's functions will have a negative effect on the thyroid. These inner functional relationships are true of all three embryological systems.

It's important to understand that all of our organs function as integrated systems. Not one tissue or organ contains cells that work independently of cells in other tissues and organs. The cells in a particular tissue support and are supported by cells in other tissues. In other words, our health is dependent upon the well-being and stable functioning of our organ and tissue *systems,* not upon just the individual organs, tissues, or cells.

All of our organs belong to one of the three original embryological systems from which they were developed. For example, if we experience liver problems, it is not just the liver as an individual organ that is disturbed, but the whole endodermic system that produced the liver and the other organs that constitute the digestive system. The fact that each individual organ is in reality part of a larger system explains why natural treatments like those that use herbs are so effective. An herb or spice that one might use for the liver not only contains substances that work on the liver, but also contains substances that help and support the entire endodermic system from which the liver developed.

This is an important concept in the field of natural healing and one that conventional medicine tends to ignore. We must learn to see the body as an interconnected system of properties, energies, and functions and not as just individual parts. Machines are made up of individual parts, but a living organism lives by way of the functions occurring in its integrated tissue and organ systems.

INDIVIDUAL CONSTITUTIONS

We have all noticed that each one of us differs in some ways from others. We often respond differently than our friends, for instance, to the same emotional and physical conditions and stimuli. Some of us tend to be heavier in our body structures, some slimmer; some of us have wavy hair, some straight; some have blue eyes, some brown. These differences are part of our individual makeup called our *constitution.* There are two major factors that determine the specific makeup of the human constitution. Our genes contain specific functional energy patterns that connect us to our family and our family's genetic history. These patterns, however, are also influenced by the vast energies of the universe that move through all things and all occurrences. We can get a glimpse of what this is like if we look into a kaleidoscope and view the constantly changing and beautifully emerging patterns. Our constitution, however, while moving in these intricate patterns, never changes and is the personal foundation of our physical and psychological responses.

All constitutions are made up of the same basic functional energies, but in slightly different proportions depending on the factors that are producing the individual. Three main energy configurations serve as the foundation of the constitution. One is made up of the energies reflected primarily in the ectoderm embryological tissue system. This configuration, which we could call the *nerve component*, provides the basic energy for the whole body and for all of its functions, as well as the sensitivity of our sensory system. We could call the configuration that is connected to the mesoderm tissues the *structural component*; it provides the physical structures of the body not only with its flesh, organs, and cells, but also its rhythmical abilities that are reflected in the breathing and the heartbeat. The last constitutional configuration works within the endoderm tissue system and could be termed the *metabolic component*. It is responsible for the metabolic activities of the body like digestion and hormonal balance.

The differences between individuals reflect the different proportions of these three main constitutional configurations. For example, a person with comparatively large portions of the nerval and metabolic components will have a tendency to be more outwardly creative and intellectual. He also will be prone to nervousness and lack of grounding and will find it difficult to be restful and peaceful. Those with a larger portion of the structural and metabolic component will tend to have a more peaceful emotional life, but will not grasp abstract knowledge as well as those with more of the nerval component.

When planning therapies, it is important to consider these constitutional differences. In this book, you do not need to be specifically concerned with constitutions because the therapy suggestions work on all constitutional levels. Our reason for mentioning the constitution is in order to explain why physical and emotional responses are unique to each person.

CHAPTER 3

Health and Disease

The fields of Classical medicine such as Ayurvedic medicine, Chinese medicine, homeopathy, and European naturopathy have always questioned conventional medicine's viewpoint regarding health and disease. Central to any discussion of health and disease is the role of the immune system. Classical medical traditions interpret the role and function of the immune system quite differently from conventional medicine. As a result, the therapies of Classical medicines differ, often significantly, from those of conventional medicine.

Conventional medicine regards the immune system and its activities as one of the major mechanisms of the body's health. It describes the immune system as being composed of various physiological components that defend the body primarily against invasive microbial pathogens. For the last hundred years, the theory of microbial pathology known as the "germ theory" has been fundamental to the diagnosis and treatment of most diseases. This approach accounts for the continual development of antimicrobial medicines like vaccines, as well as antibacterial, antiviral, and antifungal drugs, which are used in the treatment of most health issues.

This perspective, however, has failed to account for a number of important points. Ninety percent of the body's cells have a microbial basis. Most of our cells contain mitochondria, which are actually related to primitive bacteria cells. The mitochondria are responsible for the cell's energy metabolism and play an important role in the life of the body. The presence of mitochondria in our cells tells us something fascinating about the life of complex beings like ourselves. In a metaphoric sense, the microbe and its functions migrated from the outer world of our environment to the inner world of our organism. This means that our body shares its primary cell functions with, and is directly connected to, the vast world of microbes that surround it and with which we share the planet. The sharing of functions and energies between organisms, such as between people and microbes, characterize one of the most important aspects of life. Just as the cosmos shares its life with the Earth, so the Earth is the flesh and blood of all its organisms. We often live under the illusion that our life is limited to what is happening inside our bodies, creating the sensation that we are separate and independent from everything else. Yet our bodies and their functions completely depend on the myriad functions of the Earth around us and the cosmos beyond. In a sense, we are one body living and sharing life in common. When we use antibiotics, we not only threaten bacterial mitochondria in our own cells and the digestive bacteria in our intestines, which is essential for our health, but we also threaten bacteria in the environment, which is essential to the health of the Earth.

We must ask ourselves, then, is the immune system primarily a defense against microbes? If its role is to destroy microbes, then why do we depend so heavily on invasive antimicrobial drugs that all have serious side effects? Is the immune system so often incapable of doing its job? Or is there an overlooked relationship between stress, which affects the mind and body, and the immune system? Furthermore, what role do toxins play in the function of the immune system?

THE IMMUNE SYSTEM AS INTEGRATION SYSTEM

Classical medicine regards the immune system not as a defense mechanism but as an *integration system*. It recognizes that each of the major organ systems contributes to specific aspects of general immunity and that immunity depends on the function of the body as a whole, rather than on any one specific set of physiological or biochemical components. Classical medicine also recognizes that the mind not only affects the immune system and its functions but has immune processes of its own that work in much the same way as its physiological counterparts. After all, for true health, do we need to defend ourselves against life or do we need to learn to integrate and live in harmony with all the aspects of life?

Simply stated, when we look at life, we see that a vast number of influences surround us, influences that also surround and affect all of nature. These influences include everything from climate to microbes to the activities of plants, animals, and humans, and all of the events that occur between. Health is a matter of being able to relate to and integrate these influences. Whenever we cannot integrate a particular aspect of our world, our immune system will react in order to help us restore harmony to body and mind.

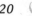

HEALTH AND THE DISEASE PROCESS

In our culture's conventional way of practicing medicine, we make a distinction between being sick and being healthy, between disease and health. In essence, we mean that disease is the *opposite* of health and that disease endangers the healthy functions of our body and mind. When we're sick, we're not healthy; we have to combat the disease to regain our health. We are so used to perceiving things this way that we never stop to ask ourselves, What is the true nature of what we call "disease"? Does nature have a purpose for disease that extends beyond just making us sick?

All living organisms contain and experience disease as part of living. Life is a process that includes disease as an integral part of its progression from birth to death. One way of responding to this fact is to view life as dangerous and full of diseases lurking around every corner. As a consequence of this perspective, we must prepare to defend our lives and fight for our health. This viewpoint parallels other cultural themes within our society, such as politics and conventional medicine, where we need to aggressively defend ourselves from continual threat.

Interestingly, when we observe domesticated animals and pets, we notice that when they are sick, they show no fear but seem to deal with pain and discomfort without agitation, instinctively knowing that what they are going through is a normal process in their lives. They only show true fear when directly threatened. We humans, on the other hand, often exude fear, agitation, and worry when sick. Except in clearly life-threatening circumstances, this is not an intuitive or instinctual reaction that is in keeping with the reality of the situation, but a projection of our cultural assumptions regarding natural disease processes. We have learned that disease is always a threat and that it is contrary to the natural order.

Classical science challenges our assumptions regarding the nature of health and the role that disease plays in the life of our organism. The word *health* stems from an old English word meaning "whole" and "holy." The concept of disease is not the opposite of the concept of health. There is no opposite of "whole" or "holy." Disease cannot make you not-whole or not-holy, because both disease and health occur within the whole person. Disease is not the *enemy* of health but is an *essential part* of the dynamic nature of health itself.

Thus, we see that no real distinction exists between "health" and "disease." Health is not the *opposite* of disease, but *contains* it. In Classical medicine, disease is understood as being one of the main ways in which the mind and body evolve. Disease, then, contributes to our growth and development. It is considered a form of natural inner medicine that creates changes in the patterns of our lives, patterns that ultimately need changing.

Nothing in life is at a standstill; everything continually moves forward, developing and evolving. Life pulls us forward into itself, exchanging new and better means of responding to patterns that no longer enhance our development. Disease is one of the processes by which the mind and body move forward and unfold into greater and greater potentials. An old European term that means "disease" is *Afflictio Divina,* which means "divine affliction." This term acknowledges that in the divine order disease exists for our own good, not as a punishment but as a way for us to grow and mature into our full personal potentials.

Tibetan and Ayurvedic medicines often call disease an "elixir," meaning a remedy or medicine that promotes our health. Therapy is not seen as combating disease, but as *cooperating* with its insistence for growth and change. In Classical medical traditions, therapeutic remedies like herbs or minerals support the inner healing and evolutionary processes initiated by disease. They enable the body to better evolve through and integrate the changes initiated by the disease for the purpose of enhancing our health and wholeness.

Classical medicine teaches that all diseases have their origin in only two fundamental causes: *lack of respect for the laws of nature* and *ignorance.* Lack of respect means that we feel that we're above the laws by which nature governs itself. This attitude affects the way we live our daily lives and moves us away from the wholeness/healthfulness that is the definition and reality of nature, the same nature that we are a part of and entirely dependent upon. We feel that we can bypass natural laws and processes, and manipulate and control nature rather than cooperating and being a part of it.

Ignorance means that we have not informed ourselves about those laws of nature that contain and reflect wholeness and health. Perhaps we have chosen not to inform ourselves or perhaps the knowledge is difficult to attain within the limits of our society. Regardless, this lack of knowledge affects the decisions we make about our lifestyles. It may cause us, for instance, to use an antibiotic on a simple symptom, even though antibiotics do not follow the natural laws of causes, symptoms, or healing processes. If this lack of knowledge did not influence our choices, we would instead use a substance, such as an herb, that *contains* in its own organism the natural laws and the mechanisms of healing that we need.

Symptoms of disease are part of the body's specialized language. They tell us that something important needs attention, that something needs changing so we can live more fully. We need to stop doing *that* and start doing *this* in order to be more aware of and experience more deeply the love, care, and continual unfolding of life. If we resist such change and ignore the language of symptoms, their meaning, and what they are trying to accomplish, we have lost a tremendous opportunity to enhance our experience of wholeness/health and personal growth.

Health is in reality an *attitude* about life. It is the way we choose to behave and respond to the infinite movement of life in and around us. Our choices all have consequences. We experience our true wholeness and health by gaining an unconditional awe and respect for life. We do this by becoming more intimate with life as we search for insight and clarity within its boundless relationships.

CHAPTER 4

Symptoms and Causes of Disease

An essential approach to curing the body is understanding the difference between a *symptom* and a *cause*. All observable symptoms in the body are caused by one or more factors. Symptoms are *never* causes and causes are *never* symptoms. If you have irritable bowel syndrome, for example, the symptoms may include pain in the bowels and mucus-coated or bloody stools. These symptoms did not appear spontaneously. Some set of factors *caused* the bowels to react like this. Thus, in order to cure the disease, we have to find the factors that are causing the symptoms and resolve them rather than just *suppressing* the symptoms through chemical medicines. In studies of this condition, conventional medicine has admitted that up to 60 percent of all irritable bowel symptoms are caused by psychological stresses. Yet, all drugs prescribed for this condition focus only on the tissues of the bowel itself and ignore treating the psychological causes.

When dealing with health issues, we need to understand the nature of symptoms. A symptom, like a runny nose or sore throat, is the body's response to some factor or group of factors. It is not really a disease. A fever doesn't just suddenly appear without any reason but is the body's response to some condition that needs attention. The body *creates* fever as part of the solution.

Symptoms are the language of the body and communicate to us the processes that it is undergoing. To better comprehend why the body does what it does and why it creates symptoms, we need only use our common sense to clearly discern the patterns in nature that mirror life, health, and disease. Let's look at the example of a tree. In the spring and summer, when the life force is strongest, the tissues of the tree fill with fluids that rise throughout the whole organism, filling the leaves with life-giving sap and making them sensitive to receiving the heat and light of the sun in order to grow and develop. During these seasons, everything in nature fills with moisture and heat.

In the fall and winter, the leaves die. When we pick up a dead leaf, we see that it is dry, brittle, and cold, whereas the living leaf was moist and supple and responded to light and heat. If we carefully consider our observations, we can learn something very important about health and the body. The greatest noticeable difference between the live leaf and the dead leaf—between life and death—involves the ability to create *moisture* and *fluids* and react to *warmth*. All living organisms have the capacity to create and use fluids and to transform nutrients. This transformation is done through metabolism, a process involving *heat*. The ability of an organism to nourish itself, to grow, and maintain its health depends on the biological heat of life working in the fluid environment of the organism.

COLD PHASE AND HOT PHASE

According to the Classical medical traditions, the factors that create disease are the factors that produce coldness, dryness, brittleness, and irregular or inhibited functions in the body-mind's living processes. As in the example of the leaf, the lack of moisture and heat indicate that it can no longer sustain life. The reduction of biological heat and moisture are factors that cause functional disturbances in cells, leading eventually to death. The lack of heat and moisture is called the *Cold Phase* of the health issue. The Cold Phase contains all the factors that create true disease.

If the body's immunity is normal, the body will react to Cold Phase factors by producing a *Hot Phase* response that restores balance. When we catch a cold in the winter, it is a result of having been exposed to the climate's cold and drying energies. If these factors are not quickly resolved, our bodies will respond by going into a Hot Phase. We may then experience fever and more activity in the fluids of the mucous membranes. This response underscores our body's ability to restore the balance of its biological heat and moisture.

If the body's immune system is compromised and is in what we call a state of low immunity or immune deficiency, the body will not be able to rebalance its biological functions with a Hot Phase reaction. As a result, the Cold Phase will become chronic and will continue to drain and damage the life of the body, producing degenerative diseases such as multiple sclerosis, cancer, and osteoarthritis.

We can easily recognize acute Cold Phase factors. They include feeling chilled or tired, having a decreased appetite, weak digestion, anxiety, and stress, and seeking comfort for the body and mind. The causes of an acute Cold Phase include getting chilled in a draft or cold, fright, anxiety, stress, overwork, overcrowded conditions, mild food poisoning, unhealthy diet, overexertion, overexercise, too much heat from the sun (which dries), and exposure to toxins, poisons, and medicines.

When the Cold Phase aspects are not resolved by Hot Phase responses and then become chronic, the following symptoms can often be observed: a general feeling of uneasiness, an inability to be pleased by the things that are usually pleasurable, lack of a sense of humor, feeling depressed, sleep troubles (can't fall asleep, wake soon after falling asleep), chronic cold hands and feet (not due to the weather), chronic irregularity like constipation, irregular menses, lack of appetite, lethargy, and lack of inspiration or enthusiasm. When healthy, our immune systems will always produce a quick response to the Cold Phase factors that endanger our health by producing a Hot Phase reaction. Again, these responses are not diseases but ways in which our immune system counteracts the Cold Phase factors that damage our body's health.

It is easy to identify Hot Phase healing factors. They are: fever, swelling, mucus, inflammation or feeling of heat in body, restlessness, nausea, sleep disturbance (wake at 3 am to 4 am), and intermittent feverish sleep. In addition, the acute phase usually involves bacteria, yeast, or viral activity as part of the healing process. These Hot Phase reactions transport heat and fluids to our cells and tissues. The heat, like that present in fever, accelerates metabolism in our tissues in order to cleanse and resolve their impaired condition. Swelling transports vital fluids containing nutrients and immune substances to our tissues. When mucous membranes react efficiently, they cleanse tissues by producing different kinds of phlegm.

COLD PHASES, HOT PHASES, AND MICROBES

Viruses, bacteria, and yeast microorganisms help tissues repair themselves. These microorganisms don't *cause* normal colds or flu, earaches, or sore throats, but only appear as part of the immune response *after* the factors involved in the Cold Phase have had a damaging influence on the body's ability to maintain its balance. Conventional medicine uses the "exposure theory" when describing conditions like colds and influenza. It claims that you become sick when exposed to the virus or bacteria that other people, who may be considered contagious, have. It's interesting to note, however, that statistically no more than 30 to 40 percent of any group known to be exposed to influenza will actually get the flu. What about those who were exposed but didn't contract it? If they all were exposed and the virus was the main cause, then the virus would infect them all. Conventional medicine has never been able to explain this anomaly.

Both Classical traditions as well as some modern Western medical research refer to microbial activity as taking place in what is called the *terrain*. What they mean by this term is that microbes only become active in the sense of producing symptoms when the conditions of the terrain are right. The exposure theory is weak in that if the microbes cause disease, everyone exposed would be infected yet we know that this is not the case. The terrain theory explains that only the individuals who share the same vulnerabilities in their own inner terrain experience the symptoms.

To give an example of the terrain mechanism, we could say that in a school class of twenty children, one comes down with the flu, then several more children catch it. By the time the flu has run itself out, less than half the class has caught the flu, even though all were exposed to it. The children who caught the flu shared certain circumstances of terrain with one another, while the others who didn't catch the flu did not share these same inner factors. These conditions involve terrain factors that lower immunity and the individual's ability to integrate their current circumstances. Factors may include an unhealthy diet, physical or emotional stress at home or in school, chronic low immunity from vaccines or prescription/nonprescription drugs, toxins in the environment, lack of sufficient rest, worry or anxiety, too much emotional stimulation from television, and overextending the body in sports activities.

The concept of terrain is based on the ability of the individual to integrate the circumstances that surround them. We must remember that the immune system is really an integration system that allows the body to respond and deal with whatever it comes into contact. The children in the school classroom who have a healthy lifestyle and can integrate the stressors of their home and school life did not get the flu. The ones who contracted the flu were in a Cold Phase pattern, which was followed by a Hot Phase healing response. Remember that microbes are part of the healing process because they stimulate an immune response.

To further illustrate this concept of Cold and Hot Phases, the terrain, and immune responses where microbes play a role, we can use the example of more extreme Cold Phase diseases. Chronic Cold Phase issues ultimately create degeneration in the organ and tissue systems of the body and result in diseases such as cancer and multiple sclerosis. These cases have one thing in common: the patient almost invariably says, "I don't understand why I have this serious disease. I haven't been sick for twenty years! When there is flu going around the office, I never get it. I thought I was so healthy." In reality, this statement indicates that the person was in a chronic Cold Phase where the immune system was so low that it couldn't create the Hot Phase of even simple healing processes that would resolve the Cold Phase influences.

The Cold Phase is degenerative and doesn't have any of the acute symptoms that the Hot Phase does. We misinterpret symptoms (or the lack thereof) and assume that the Hot Phase with its symptoms *is* the disease, whereas, in fact, it is the *healing process*. The Hot Phase is an immune process that shows the immune system is active and doing what it should to heal the body from Cold Phase factors. If the Hot Phase immune responses do not resolve the Cold Phase factors, the Cold Phase becomes chronic and systemic. This indicates an immune deficiency, which means that the immune system will not be able to respond well in the ongoing healing mode responsible for continually balancing and integrating our body-mind functions. When the immune system is low, the degenerative processes that create serious diseases will continue to progress slowly to the point where they finally become visible in symptoms such as tumors or serious organ dysfunction.

COLD AND HOT PHASES AND THE MIND

According to Classical medicine, because the mind is connected directly to bodily functions, it, too, experiences Cold and Hot Phase processes. An example of a chronic mental Cold Phase pattern is depression. Depression is degenerative in the sense that it is a closing down or lack of emotional/mental response to the circumstances facing us. Often one of the first indications that depression is starting to heal is the manifestation of a Hot Phase. Examples of mental Hot Phase reactions include anger and irritation. Like fever, swelling, and mucous symptoms in the body's Hot Phase response, anger and irritation are hot, strong, and focused reactions to circumstances. As the original causes of the mental issues are resolved, anger and irritation disappear in the same way that fever resolves itself.

The key point to remember is that the immune system, in its job of integrating all of our mental and physical issues, *is always giving the best possible response it can to any given circumstance at any given time*. The only way we can increase the immune system's abilities to keep us in balance and deal with the factors that affect our health is to create a healthy lifestyle and support the immune system through proper natural healing methods.

CHAPTER 5

The Whole Person

All medical traditions have in some way dealt with the concept that man is a whole being made up of body, soul, and spirit. Classical medicine attempts to take these three important aspects of our lives into consideration when evaluating health and disease processes. In addition, it describes the nature and role of the psyche, the soul, and the spirit, and explains how each of these relate to the functions of the body. It has become popular to refer to the human organism as being a mind-body entity, an indication that we are beginning to comprehend that our lives are not merely physical or chemical processes, but intimately involve the psyche, soul, and spirit.

THE EMBRYOLOGICAL TISSUE SYSTEMS AND THE MIND

As previously discussed, our mind and its emotions are directly connected to the functions of our body's organs. Because all organs are developed from one of the three embryological systems, these systems play as significant a role in our mental health as in our physical health. A number of parts of our anatomy contain "reflex maps" of all our organs and tissue functions. When certain parts of the body are compromised, these areas reflect the compromising factors by undergoing subtle changes in their tissues. They also may develop a greater susceptibility to pain in specific points that respond to the systems of the body being compromised. We can find these reflex maps of our body in the iris of the eye, the inner nasal passages, the outer ear, the feet, and the hands. Natural medical practices often make use of these reflex points in therapies like reflexology, ear acupuncture, and iris diagnosis.

The brain is another of these reflex maps. The embryological tissue systems each have their own brain reflex area. Each specific brain area is connected to a particular embryological organ and its tissues. When an organ or tissue of the body becomes diseased or functionally compromised, a specific area of the brain undergoes subtle changes. Research carried out through photo imaging of the brain has been able to map the connection between brain tissue responses and health issues in the organ systems.

In the brain, the ectoderm is reflected in the nerve tissues of the cerebral cortex (large brain bark). The ectoderm system and the large brain bark are very sensitive to emotional conflicts that have to do with territory. The territorial relationships that exist in our home, work, or school environment have emotional components. When we feel that the relationships or events occurring in our territory threaten our physical or mental well-being, we can develop a territorial conflict that compromises the organs and tissues of the ectoderm system as well as its reflex, the large brain bark. Territorial conflict can lead to diseases of the nerve system or to changes in our emotional behavior. Often, we either try to shrink into the background in order to escape a perceived threat or we become aggressive in an effort to overcome the threat. We may attempt to create a persona who will fit in, a persona we can show to our parents or our boss, while our own true personality remains safely hidden. Such responses allow the mind to compensate for the stress it is experiencing in its territory. Though these compensating mechanisms seem to work, they don't really solve the problem. Symptoms of the conflict can develop in the tissues associated with the ectoderm, creating symptoms in the skin, hair, or nails, or result in nerve tension that affects tissues in various parts of the body.

The endoderm is reflected in the medulla oblongata (the brain stem). The endoderm system and its reflex to the brain stem are sensitive to what we call "nutritional" conflicts. We must remember in this context that our lives are nurtured by spiritual, mental, and emotional, as well as physical sources. The tissues and organs responsible for our digestion and metabolism can be compromised by conflicts in any of the areas that nurture us. Nutritional conflicts are relatively easy to understand: either we're getting too much of something, too little of something, or we can't digest what we're getting and therefore it isn't right for us. When we say "I have too much responsibility," "I have too much work," "I just don't have enough time for myself," or "I can't find the things that really relax me," "I should never have chosen to do this," and "It's just not me and it's dragging me down," we express nutritional conflicts. Physically, nutritional conflicts are seen in the vomiting reflex, diarrhea, constipation, continual hunger, weight loss, weight gain, being unsatisfied by eating, and feeling heavy, tired, or overly full after eating.

In the mesoderm system, the brain reflexes are the cerebral medulla (large brain marrow) and the cerebellum (small brain). These brain areas control the inner integrating functions of the body and mind. They act as a communication center for coordinating the signals conveyed by the nerve system to all organs and their tissues, as well as to the muscle/skeletal system and the digestive processes. They also reflect deeper aspects of our psychological identity and react to conflicts involving our self-esteem and self-worth. Whenever we feel that our integrity is being attacked, when we feel wounded by someone's opinion of us, or feel personally unworthy and suffer from lack of self-esteem, the organs and tissues that originate in the mesoderm will be affected. Our heart and circulatory system, bones, joints, and muscles, along with the makeup and function of our blood can become diseased or functionally disturbed.

Figure 5.1 will help you understand how the body and mind function as interrelated systems. The figure eight shows how the systems are dynamically related. Imagine that the figure is like a circle twisted over on itself to form two loops joined in the center. The loop constantly moves so that the energies of the top loop travel down into the bottom loop by passing through the center point. The movement of the figure shows how the energies and qualities of the specific areas of the body and mind influence one another. The top loop eventually creates the bottom loop as the bottom loop eventually creates the top loop. Both pass through the center point, which works as a balancing factor between the two loops.

THE ACTIVITY OF THE PSYCHE

The *psyche* is the invisible organ of our emotions. It reflects all our feelings, such as fear, depression, joy, and anxiety. We tend to believe that our feelings are based on what is happening to us at any given moment, whereas in reality they also reflect how we are functioning on deeper physical levels. This occurs because the functions of the psyche are directly connected to the functions of the body's organ systems.

In Classical medicine, we see that each organ system controls a portion of the processes reflecting our emotional responses. For instance, when the Kidney System is not functioning optimally and is unable to integrate our experiences, chronic anxiety can result. The feeling of fear can be produced by low blood sugar, as well as chronic constipation. Anger, irritability, and depression are connected to the functions of the Liver/Gallbladder System, while worry is a reflection of functions in the spleen, stomach, and pancreas; sorrow and grief reflect the functions of our lungs.

The direct connections between the psyche and the body underline why a

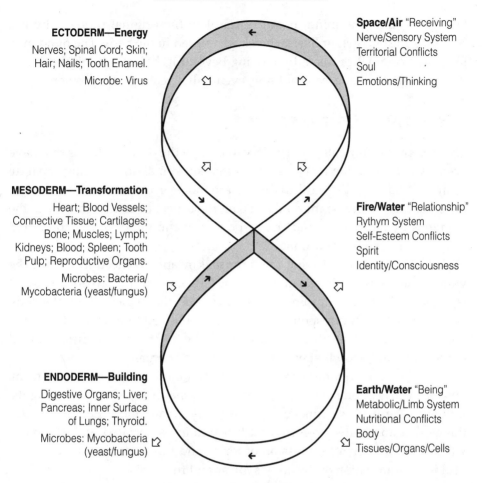

ECTODERM—Energy

Nerves; Spinal Cord; Skin;
Hair; Nails; Tooth Enamel.

Microbe: Virus

Space/Air "Receiving"
Nerve/Sensory System
Territorial Conflicts
Soul
Emotions/Thinking

MESODERM—Transformation

Heart; Blood Vessels;
Connective Tissue; Cartilages;
Bone; Muscles; Lymph;
Kidneys; Blood; Spleen; Tooth
Pulp; Reproductive Organs.

Microbes: Bacteria/
Mycobacteria (yeast/fungus)

Fire/Water "Relationship"
Rythym System
Self-Esteem Conflicts
Spirit
Identity/Consciousness

ENDODERM—Building

Digestive Organs; Liver;
Pancreas; Inner Surface
of Lungs; Thyroid.

Microbes: Mycobacteria
(yeast/fungus)

Earth/Water "Being"
Metabolic/Limb System
Nutritional Conflicts
Body
Tissues/Organs/Cells

Figure 5.1. "The Figure Eight"

therapist can address issues in the psyche and the emotions through a treatment such as acupuncture, which restores the proper functioning of the organ systems. It's hard for many to understand that sticking a small acupuncture needle in a specific point on the skin can decrease depression, sorrow, irritability, and other emotions by reestablishing the energies of an organ system.

If these emotions remain unresolved, they linger as tension in their specific tissue systems. This tension continually stimulates and reproduces the original emotion, making the trauma very difficult to heal. Psychological counseling alone can be of benefit *only* if it resolves the emotion *and* releases the tension. Often, because standard psychological counseling does not treat the body as well as the mind, it can restimulate the original problem by not resolving the energetic-physical blockages stored in the body. The mind may forget the original problem by moving beyond it, but certain physical dysfunctions and tensions can continue, eventually creating new problems.

THE ACTIVITY OF THE SOUL

The soul can be difficult to define because of all the different terms that have been used to describe it. The soul is often spoken about as being separate from the body. All Classical traditions are more precise about the nature of the soul. They describe the soul as being the aspect of us that integrates the emotions of the psyche and the responses of the mind and is connected directly to the body's functions.

To better understand what the term *soul* means, we need to look at the word in the original Greek language. The Greek word for soul is *animus* and is found in the root of our English word *animate,* that which allows the body and mind to live and respond. Animus is traditionally understood as being the "breath of life," a collective term for all the functional energies involved in the mind and body that make up the life of our organism.

Thoughts and emotions share one thing in common: they each have form. Spoken words, along with the words that come in the shape of thoughts, influence the way we function because they create and reflect forms. All things that are related to form and function are associated with the body, which itself is a living expression of forms and functions. In this sense, the soul is the foundation of the body's forms and functions.

THE SPIRIT AND CONSCIOUSNESS

The teachings of Classical medicine always includes a discussion of the spirit and consciousness. Our mind has two different dimensions. One of these is the ability to think, feel, and express itself through the forms of thought, language, and emotion. The other dimension of the mind is what we call consciousness. Consciousness itself does not contain or produce forms and is therefore considered the realm of the spirit, which embraces all things.

Our consciousness does not "think" thoughts, nor does it have any emotions, but rather is a kind of *pure and clear awareness* that is always present in the background of all processes taking place in the body and soul. Like a mirror, the consciousness of spirit reflects life in all of its dimensions and connects us directly to all that exists. All traditions consider the spirit to be the organ of communication between the divine and the body and soul. Consciousness, therefore, is associated with wisdom, with our ability to understand and experience the universal principles and the events of life on a deep intuitive level instead of just acquiring knowledge about them. Intellectual knowledge deals with processing thought forms; it is a dimension of the body and soul, not the spirit.

Though the spirit does not contain thought or emotions, it definitely affects our thinking and our emotions. Because of the direct connection between mind and body, the body can tense up when faced with emotional conflicts. Emotional responses are given form and relayed through the body via its organs and tissue systems. These systems tend to retain the effect of the emotions until the conflict is resolved and transformed. The consciousness of the spirit, on the other hand, helps us by engaging the conscious faculty of wisdom in order to resolve emotional issues and their effect on the body. Wisdom accompanies the activities of consciousness and provides consciousness with a far greater capacity to comprehend the larger reality behind emotional events.

We experience our consciousness when it breaks in on emotional issues that seem hopelessly tangled and stuck. Our mind is busy with the endless repetitions of "what if this" and "what if that" as it attempts to resolve a situation. As our consciousness sheds light into this tangle of contradicting emotions, we suddenly understand things in a new way. This unexpected clarity brings healing to the emotional issues. This is why the traditions of prayer, contemplation, creativity, and meditation—all activities that engage the consciousness and wisdom of the spirit—play an essential role in our physical and mental health.

THE CHALLENGE OF DEATH

The most challenging aspect of life that we face is death. Our culture tends to define death as the opposite and enemy of life, just as it defines disease as the opposite and the enemy of health. Death is seen as the end result of disease or a failure in one or more of the body's "parts." In the past, our understanding of death came mainly from the spiritual insights and teachings of our religious institutions and communities. More recently, our knowledge and attitude regarding death has been influenced by the uncertainty, inability, and reluctance of the scientific community to involve itself in the discussion.

Classical medical sciences approach the subject of death quite differently. Classical doctors begin their training and teachings with what we would call the spiritual foundations of life. These health sciences do not define death as the opposite of life nor as its enemy. Rather, they say that life *contains* death, just as health *contains* disease. Life is an absolute that by definition has no opposite—there is no dead life, nor live death—only life in a continual and creative state of transition and transformation.

Death is always a servant to life and is the way that life shapes space and time. Every second, thousands of cells die in our body in order to make room for new, more vital cells; one thought dies and gives way to another so that we experience and learn. Life continually expands and creates new ways of expressing itself. Our childhood response patterns die and their death becomes the foundation upon which adulthood builds itself in the ongoing search for new ways to experience and express life. Our memories are the forms of things experienced in the past that we bring into our present moments, where together the past and present are shaped into new experiences. Life never loses anything; it builds forward from within with greater and greater abilities to experience and express itself.

Death is one of the means by which life transforms and renews itself. All things and moments in time and space change and are in a constant transition that does not challenge the *absolute* nature of life, but *enhances* it. Paradoxically, we accept the changes that involve death, such as those that occur during the transitional phases of puberty when the response patterns of childhood die and reemerge as new experiences that affirm life anew. Yet, we struggle in great anxiety when faced with the fact of dying in the transition that involves the death of our body. Our spiritual nature and its intuitive knowledge, however, challenge the idea that life is defined *solely* by its biological processes. We are life incarnate, born from life into life, and are constantly transforming from within in its endless ability to express and affirm itself. Even the humble process of digestion illustrates death becoming life. Through the death and transformation process that food undergoes in our digestive system, our bodies build and sustain new life.

The spiritual teachings of all religions and traditions claim that death is not only a part of life, but that death cannot define nor diminish life. They state, each in their own way, that life is an absolute that has an eternal dimension. Even seemingly different concepts, such as the Eastern perspectives of reincarnation and the Christian/Judaic/Islamic concept regarding the eternal nature of the Self, agree that death is a transition that occurs within life and that life is an absolute that can never be diminished by death, only expanded.

The Classical medical sciences have maintained and made use of these concepts regarding life, health, and death, whereas our culture has separated the spiritual knowledge that deals with these issues from the more mechanistic philosophy that dominates conventional medicine. To be fully alive and to be truly healthy, we need to better understand the role of death and dying in the processes of life. We need to stop thinking in opposites and start thinking in wholes, embracing the life that defines the reality within which we live.

Spiritual knowledge comes not from being able to weigh and measure things, which is what our science relies upon, but through the knowledge and wisdom that resides in our deepest consciousness. Our consciousness tells us that life is far greater than its parts and has dimensions that are absolute even though, like love, they can't be reproduced in a scientific experiment. Intuitively we know that science is a tool not a source of absolute knowledge, yet we often give our sciences an authority over all other forms of knowledge and rely on them to provide the facts upon which we base our lives. This limitation can reduce our lives to a death waiting to happen, an anxiety that hides like a subtle darkness behind our pleasures and hopes and stifles creative participation in our own daily lives.

The death we fear—the final and permanent negation of the loves, hopes, and dreams that a person has lived and strived for and the cruel end to the nobility of Self—is an impossibility. The death we fear is a mysterious paradox that goes against everything our inner self knows. Death is a transition and transformation process, like all other processes in life, and it can only serve life, not conquer or destroy it.

This concept is hard for us to readily accept because we have been brought up in the machine-technology culture of medicine and we fear the failure of the machine, our body, when it will no longer function as it used to. We seem to be caught in this broken machine concept of death because we are no longer in contact with the deeper knowledge of the consciousness that is distilled into the teachings of the great religions. We tend to reject the validity of any concept that is not verifiable through our sciences and in doing so we have replaced an illuminated consciousness with an analytical abstraction.

HEALING: A REFLECTION OF THE WHOLE PERSON

You might ask at this point, "What does all of this have to do with health?" Consider this: we are all made up of what we call body, mind, and spirit. These three dimensions are tied together in a single unity called "me"—the body with its energetic and biological processes; the mind with its mental and emotional capacities; and the spirit with its deep consciousness. We are more or less familiar with the body and its processes and are aware of our emotional lives to some degree, but many of us remain unfamiliar with the all-embracing activities and lessons of consciousness.

Health concerns the whole of us, not just a part. We give the body a great amount of attention, ranging from diets, fitness plans, and beauty treatments to medical and alternative therapies. We consult doctors, psychiatrists, and psychotherapists to deal with the mind. But few of us give daily attention to the care and nourishment of the spirit. We seem to forget that our spiritual needs are as great as those of the body and, if we neglect them, the consequences will affect our health, just as if we neglected the needs of the body.

In Classical medical practice, a consultation for any health issue typically includes dietary changes and natural therapies to support and enhance the body's healing processes; instructions on behavioral changes that modify and support the healing of the mind and emotions; and directives involving spiritual practices that support the healing process of the whole person.

Today, our Western societies are infused with so many different cultures that it would be inappropriate to prescribe any one particular spiritual path or regimen for health. Doctors and therapists from different health systems, however, should advise everyone to be active and conscientious about their spiritual lives. After all, the term *holistic medicine* is precisely that—a practice that works with the whole person, not just his or her separate parts.

CHAPTER 6

The Language of Science in Medical Models

Our word *science* comes from the Latin root *scire*, which means "to know." All traditions of medicine are based on science, the way of "knowing" things. Each tradition has developed its own methods of knowing along with a language that conveys this knowledge and is compatible with its culture and practices.

We are most familiar with the way in which Western science knows things and the language it uses to express this knowledge. Our scientific methods are called *reductionist methods* because we base our knowledge of the world on a science of matter. The research methods of conventional medicine take things apart, reducing them to smaller and smaller components. The history of this medical science began with the discovery of the organs, then reduced them down to tissues, then to cells, and finally to their chemical compounds, DNA, and genes. This science is based on the belief that we can best understand how something works by discovering its parts and seeing how they fit with one another in order to function. This approach comes from the trend of technological development that has been the major characteristic of our culture for the last two centuries. A technological view of the world tends to consider the universe as something mechanical that is made up of and functions by way of its parts. Our scientific language and its methods identify and describe these parts.

The sciences of other cultures are not based on this same belief system. They rely on other means of knowing and use different words and images to describe and define what they know. Though their languages sound strange to us at first, the scientific systems of other cultures are just as valid as our systems. Classical medical sciences are more concerned with describing how things function not by their parts, but by identifying the universal forces and natural laws that determine their function. When a Chinese doctor speaks of Kidney ch'i, an energy that enables and determines the functions of the kidney, he is not using the language of Western science that speaks of cells and chemical activities. He is instead referring to a form of biological energy that can't be weighed or measured through the instrumentation of conventional medicine. A potential conflict arises between these two medical sciences in that conventional medicine insists upon being able to isolate, weigh, and measure things if they are to be acceptable to their science. The potential confusion that derives from this difference in approach increases due to the language of Classical medicine, which uses metaphors to describe the nature of the body's systems and their functions.

SCIENTIFIC METAPHORS

Scientific metaphors do not describe the parts of matter but rather describe the fundamental, universal forces that determine their qualities and activities. In this sense, Classical medicine believes that knowing about and understanding these forces—what they mean, how they act, and how they determine the functions of bodily systems—is more important than knowing about the parts that make up an organ's structure, such as its cells or the chemicals it produces.

Metaphors prove very useful in science because the forces and qualities they describe are universal properties shared by all things and all events. Thus, metaphors allow us to connect the function of things with their specific properties and activities, properties that are shared by all other events occurring in nature. By making these connections, we can develop a picture of how things work and how they are all interrelated.

The metaphoric language of classical science and the parts-and-pieces language of Western science are not really contradictory but complementary. Both have contributed significantly to medical science. Whenever strong and immediate intervention is necessary, such as in the event of a severe trauma, Western science excels because it understands how to replace, diminish, and block one function with another through its knowledge of cellular chemistry. In understanding the disease process and how to return the body to its normal functions, Classical medicine excels with its knowledge of how the body works as an integrated set of systems and the how biological energies of these systems control the body's processes and maintain its health.

Most recently, these two traditions have found a meeting place in the science of quantum physics. The Western science of quantum physics has discovered that the perspectives of the classical sciences have great validity. Quantum physics does not view the universe as being made up of parts but understands that it functions by way of dynamic energy patterns that have an ever-changing effect on the forms and functions of all matter. Applied to the field of medicine, it is these dynamic universal energies that determine the functions of cells, tissues, and organs and their biochemical reactions. This brings us back to the concepts and language of the classical sciences.

THE FIVE ELEMENTS

If you recall, all Classical medical traditions use metaphoric language or "images" to describe the qualities in events and how things work. One set of metaphoric images found in Classical medicine is the concept of the Elements. Elements are not things; rather they are descriptions of *qualities* and *events* that are inherent in nature and are the forces that shape and determine how things function. In this sense, the Elements describe the fundamental energy patterns of the universe. The following is an example of the Five Elements as seen by Classical medicine. By relating these descriptions to the embryological organs and tissues, you will discover some interesting connections concerning the functions of the body and mind.

In the original texts of Classical medicine, the teachings were often written in poetic language that may seem difficult to comprehend at first. Wisdom permeates this language, however, especially when we consider that metaphors describe the very dynamic and universal forces that shape and create the events and functions of life. Just as a painting or a poem often reveals something new and essential about life, so the metaphors and language of classical science reveal the mechanisms and relationships upon which life is based. We must remember that science means "seeing," not just seeing with our eyes and our instruments, but seeing with our minds and hearts as well.

The Element of Space

Listen to the silence. You can hear it in the little pause of calm stillness between your every word. It is the emptiness and space out of which all things arise. It carries you; you are surrounded by it and are immersed in it. This space contains all that occurs, will occur, and has occurred. It is the place that holds all things. It is the womb of time and matter, the container from which all things emerge and makes all things possible; the place where all things can be conceived, grow, and develop. It resists nothing and can therefore hold all things and conceive of all things. It is the birthplace of the energies that are the life of the universe. The Space Element is represented by the ear and hearing. It is active in all three embryological tissues.

The Element of Air

In the all-embracing container of Space, there are stirrings and yearnings for becoming, for creation is filled with divine presence and the irresistible desire for being, which is the origin of all forms and events. This Element is full of the whisperings and callings to become form and event, to be born out of the vastness of the universe. It invites us to reach out for life with both hands, with a willingness to receive all that life brings us. Reaching out to life and its intention to be is our first and most important step in becoming Self. It is the impulse to create and be created, not by making, but by *receiving*—to fulfill one's destiny as body among other bodies, as identity among other identities. We must allow ourselves to be created by life before we can create life ourselves. The Air Element is the *primary energy of life,* which makes it possible for all things to move and function. It is the energy behind growth and change. The Air Element is represented by the hands and touching. It is mostly associated with the ectoderm embryological tissues.

The Element of Fire

Creativity is the alchemy of the soul. It transforms impulse to vision and impregnates the fecundity of the Space Element and the creative energies of its womb with the birth of *intention.* Like the seed with its greening power, it burns away the husk of the outer shell and reveals the essence within. It is the crucible in which the heat of our passion melts away appearances and allows the heart to be one with its vision. It is the transformation, the spirit behind seeing, hearing, touching, and the body's metabolism. It brings the light of vision, wisdom, and compassion into every act, every moment of giving and receiving, which is our spiritual, emotional, and physical foundation of life. It is the heat that makes creativity an expression of the universal, burning away the limitations of unclear and half-seen images that cloud the vision and reduce illumination to mere information. The Fire Element is represented by the heart and Self. It is mostly associated with the mesoderm and endoderm embryological tissues.

The Element of Water

The watery realm of life is its fertility, providing nourishment and growth to all that can be conceived. It is the water surrounding the infant of the womb, a slow gracefulness that brings comfort and peace to the body and mind. It is the bond of relationship and sharing that connects all forms and events throughout the universe. It is the communion, the root of communication that touches the heart with new, all-embracing life. It reveals that which is shared in common, allowing the common to reveal the universal and the universal to be revealed in the common. It touches all things, seeks all things, and joins all things in the unity of life. The Water Element is represented by the reproductive organs and fertility. It is mostly associated with the mesoderm and endoderm embryological tissues.

The Element of Earth

The Earth is the solidity of form, the way in which the swirling nebula of creation reveals its identity. It is the clay from which energy becomes matter and impulse clothes itself in being. It is the new form, the new child, that which is always unique and personal, carrying its own identity into a new way of seeing and being. Yet every new child is a continuing revelation of the whole, of that which is universally real and true. The solidity of form makes the cosmos visible. It is a new and unique way for the divine imperative to reveal life as identity, as function within form, as worthy of being. The Earth Element is represented by the digestive tract, cells, and digestion. It is mostly associated with the endoderm embryological tissues.

Take time to notice the nature and qualities of the Elements at work within and around you. You will quickly see that the Elements describe how life unfolds, functions, and maintains itself.

Therapies for Common Ailments

How to Use the Therapy Section

Part Two lists health issues by category and then symptoms. Each chapter begins with a "Teaching." In the Classical medical traditions, doctors were first and foremost considered to be teachers. It was believed that without an understanding of how the body and mind functioned and remained healthy, any therapy they prescribed would only be a temporary relief and the person would continue the habits that compromised their health. The teaching presented for each health issue will give you insight into how the body and mind function as well as how and why these functions can be disturbed and lead to health problems.

Following the teaching is a "Therapy" section. We have chosen five main types of therapy that can be used to treat health problems: homeopathic tissue salts, spices, herbs, foods, and foot reflexology. This section begins with general remedies that can be used to treat particular symptoms. The ingredients for each remedy are listed. *Use what you have.* If a remedy calls for four ingredients, one of which is the spice turmeric, for example, and you don't have turmeric, you can still prepare and use the remedy without the turmeric. Most of the ingredients you will already have at home or can easily purchase at a grocery or health food store.

The general remedies are followed by recommendations for using tissue salts, herbs and spices for specific symptoms, dietary recommendations, and foot reflexology techniques.

TISSUE SALTS

Tissue salts are very effective remedies that should be an essential part of your home medicine chest, ready to be used for many of the typical problems you may experience. Tissue salts are remedies made from the mineral salts found naturally in the blood. There are a total of twelve therapeutic tissue salts, sometimes called cell salts, because they help the cells maintain proper balance and healthy function. We can support the process of restoring health and balance during illness by taking the appropriate tissue salts.

The twelve Tissue Salts (abbreviated in parentheses and followed by their common names) are:

Calcarea fluorica (Calc. fluor.)—calcium fluoride

Calcarea phosphorica (Calc. phos.)—calcium phosphate

Calcarea sulphurica (Calc. sulph.)—calcium sulphate

Ferrum phosphoricum (Ferrum phos.)—iron phosphate

Kalium muriaticum (Kali mur.)—potassium chloride

Kalium phosphoricum (Kali phos.)—potassium phosphate

Kalium sulphuricum (Kali sulph.)—potassium sulphate

Magnesium phosphorica (Mag. phos.)—magnesium phosphate

Natrum muriaticum (Natrum mur.)—sodium chloride

Natrum phosphoricum (Natrum phos.)—sodium phosphate

Natrum sulphuricum (Natrum sulph.)—sodium sulphate

Silicea (Silicea)—silicic oxide

Sometimes you may only need one tissue salt, or you may need to take four different ones at once.

Tissue Salts can be purchased in most health food stores. They should be in the form of tablets or small pills (not liquid) and in the 6X potency (D6 in Europe). The potency is listed on the package label and usually follows the name of the salt. Often, the label will list a few symptoms that the tissue salt effectively treats. While it indeed treats those symptoms, they are not by any means a complete list. If your symptoms are not listed on the label of a particular tissue salt, but this book recommends its use, go ahead and buy it for use as described in these chapters.

The dosage for tissue salts is listed on the package; however, our instructions for the frequency of doses may differ from the package. Tissue salts should be dissolved slowly in the mouth outside of meal times. For infants, dissolve the pills or tablets in a teaspoon of water. If using a spoon to break up the tablets, make sure it is plastic and not metal.

SPICES, HERBS, AND FOODS

Spices, herbs, and foods are also recommended for helping the particular health issue or symptom being discussed. For instance, in the chapter on coughs, certain spices, herbs, and foods are appropriate for a dry cough, while others are helpful for a rattling cough. Also, near the end of each therapy section is a listing of spices, herbs, and foods for general care of the ear, eye, urinary tract, or whatever particular body system is being addressed.

Spices are some of the great healers of the plant world. You can combine them as indicated in the therapy sections as well as use them in the food you eat. Use what you have. You can vary the amounts of each spice depending on how many you're combining. Or just mix the powdered spices in a teaspoon, put them directly in your mouth on the tongue, and wash the spices down with water.

Note: Microwaves should never be used, period! Microwaves destroy the vital energies of foods, causing the body to react initially as though the foods were foreign substances. In addition, the true nutritive value of the food is greatly reduced by microwaving because the metabolic processes of digestion are dependent on the energies of the food.

If spices and herbs are recommended as a medicinal tea (standard infusion or decoction), the following formula can be used to determine how much tea to give a child aged 12 or under. First, add 12 to the child's age, then divide the child's age by this total. For example, for an 8-year-old, the formula is 12 + 8 = 20; 8 divided by 20 is 0.40. The child would need 0.40 (40 percent) of an adult dosage. An adult dosage is one cup of tea.

REFLEXOLOGY

Most of the therapy sections conclude with recommendations for foot reflexology treatment, another effective way to treat acute symptoms and support immune processes. You can use it on adults and children and in conjunction with other treatments.

All of the organs and tissues of the body are directly connected to one another through two major energy systems. One of these carries functional energies and is connected through a system of channels called "meridians" in Chinese medicine and "nadis" in Ayurvedic medicine. These channels have energy points that are used to stimulate the different functions of organs and tissues. The other major system, the one referred to in this book, is composed of nerve reflexes contained in skin and connective tissues. These are called "reflex points" (see illustrations on page 49) and are used in a therapy commonly called reflexology. Reflex points are found most easily on the foot. By stimulating the reflex points with a simple massage technique, the body will increase and stabilize the organ and tissue functions they are associated with and help the body to heal.

Use your thumb or index finger to massage the reflex points (see below). These points should be stimulated in a particular order (the reflex points and order of stimulation will be indicated on the charts in each therapy section). The reflex points may feel tender when stimulating them because of the processes going on in the body as it deals with the illness. The pressure you use should be firm, but not hard enough to cause pain. Try massaging a few points on your own foot to get the feel of it.

With adults, children, or infants, you can dip your thumb and finger in castor oil, olive oil, or other cooking oil so as not to irritate the skin of the foot. This step, however, is not required. The pressure you apply to the massage should be slow and gentle with firm circular movements, about one minute to each reflex point. With infants, use a lighter touch. After you treat each point in the series indicated in the illustration, repeat the whole treatment three times, again moving point by point. For acute situations, the treatment should last about ten minutes.

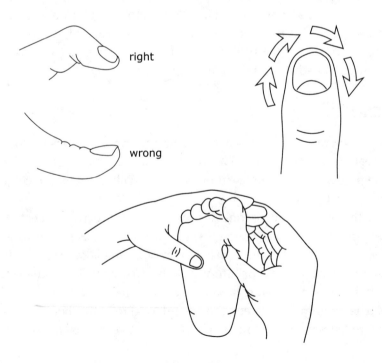

right

wrong

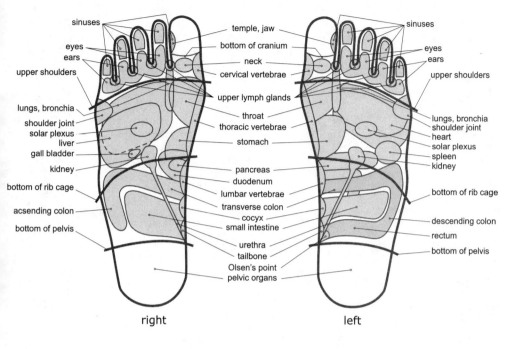

sinuses · temple, jaw · sinuses
eyes · bottom of cranium · eyes
ears · neck · ears
upper shoulders · cervical vertebrae · upper shoulders
· upper lymph glands
lungs, bronchia · throat · lungs, bronchia
shoulder joint · thoracic vertebrae · shoulder joint
solar plexus · heart
liver · stomach · solar plexus
gall bladder · spleen
kidney · pancreas · kidney
· duodenum
bottom of rib cage · lumbar vertebrae · bottom of rib cage
· transverse colon
acsending colon · cocyx · descending colon
· small intestine
bottom of pelvis · rectum
· urethra · bottom of pelvis
· tailbone
· Olsen's point
· pelvic organs

right · left

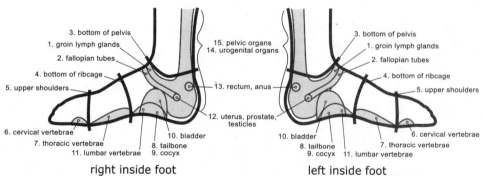

3. bottom of pelvis
1. groin lymph glands · 15. pelvic organs · 3. bottom of pelvis
2. fallopian tubes · 14. urogenital organs · 1. groin lymph glands
4. bottom of ribcage · 2. fallopian tubes
5. upper shoulders · 13. rectum, anus · 4. bottom of ribcage
· 5. upper shoulders
· 12. uterus, prostate, testicles
6. cervical vertebrae · 6. cervical vertebrae
7. thoracic vertebrae · 10. bladder · 10. bladder · 7. thoracic vertebrae
11. lumbar vertebrae · 8. tailbone · 8. tailbone · 9. cocyx · 11. lumbar vertebrae
9. cocyx

right inside foot · left inside foot

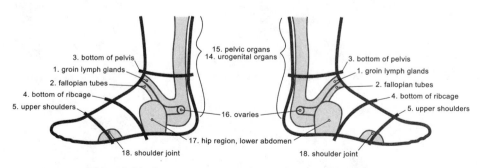

15. pelvic organs
14. urogenital organs
3. bottom of pelvis · 3. bottom of pelvis
1. groin lymph glands · 1. groin lymph glands
2. fallopian tubes · 2. fallopian tubes
4. bottom of ribcage · 4. bottom of ribcage
5. upper shoulders · 16. ovaries · 5. upper shoulders
17. hip region, lower abdomen
18. shoulder joint · 18. shoulder joint

right outside foot · left outside foot

Remedy Preparation Techniques

The following are simple and effective techniques for preparing herbal and homeopathic remedies, as well as treatments that use food.

STANDARD HOT INFUSION

Place 1 rounded teaspoon of dried herb(s) or 2 teaspoons of crushed fresh herb(s) in a cup. If using multiple herbs, divide teaspoon into parts (i.e., use $^1/_2$ teaspoon for two herbs; $^1/_4$ teaspoon for up to four herbs, for a total of 1 teaspoon). Pour 1 cup of boiling water over the herbs. Cover and steep for 15 minutes; then strain out herbs and drink.

For powdered herbs or seeds, use a scant teaspoon and crush seeds slightly before steeping.

Refrigerate extra tea in a covered container for up to two days.

STANDARD COLD INFUSION

In a pot, add one 1 part herb(s) to 20 parts water (at room temperature). This equals about 1 tablespoon per cup of water. Cover pot with a cloth. Let steep for 24 hours. Strain; press excess fluids out of the herbs and dispose of them.

Refrigerate extra tea in a covered container for up to two days.

DECOCTION

Simmer 1 part herb(s), bark, or twig in 20 parts water for 10 minutes in a covered pot. Remove from heat. Let steep for 15 minutes, then strain.

Refrigerate extra tea in a covered container for up to two days.

FRESH PLANT TINCTURE

Chop fresh herb(s). Use 1 part herb to 2 parts of pure grain alcohol, such as Everclear or Puro de Cana. Mix in a glass container. Cover and steep for fourteen days; stir gently once daily. On the last day, do not stir but strain and squeeze out fluids from the herbs. Dilute the tincture by 50 percent with distilled water. Store in a covered glass bottle up to six months. Usual dosage of tincture is 10 drops, 1–3 times daily.

DRY PLANT TINCTURE

Slightly grind 1 part dried herb(s) or bark(s) (like cinnamon). In a glass container, mix herb(s) with 5 parts pure grain alcohol, such as Everclear or Puro de Cana. Steep for fourteen days, shaking the mixture twice daily for a couple of minutes. On the last day, do not shake tincture but strain and squeeze out fluids from the herbs. Dilute the tincture by 50 percent with distilled water. Store in a covered glass bottle for up to six months. Usual dosage of tincture is 10 drops, 1–3 times daily.

COMPRESS

Place desired amount of herb(s) in a container. Pour enough boiling water on herbs to barely cover them. Steep for 2 minutes, then allow to cool. Place the cooled herbs directly on injury/treatment site and cover with a cloth to hold them in place. Change up to several times a day as needed.

Vegetable Compress

Place vegetable in a pot of boiling water. For leafy vegetables, boil 1 minute; for stalky vegetables, boil 3 minutes. Strain and allow vegetable to cool. Place cooled vegetable directly on treatment site and hold in place with cloth. Change up to 6 times per day as needed.

Fruit or Vegetable Juice Compress

For fruit juice, press juice from fruit and apply directly to injury/treatment site or soak clean cloth in juice and place directly on site. For vegetable juices, simmer vegetable(s) for 8 minutes. Allow to cool, then strain. Place cooled liquid directly on treatment site or soak clean cloth in liquid and place on site.

DRIED FRUITS

Cut up dried fruits and place in a container. Add a double amount of water; soak overnight. Simmer 10 minutes before eating.

GARLIC COMPOUND

Peel 30 garlic cloves; let cloves sit for 15 minutes before processing further. Place cloves in a blender with a little water. Using short spurts, blend until homogenized. Use 1 part of garlic compound to 20 parts water; drink two times daily. Refrigerate remaining compound for up to one week.

GARLIC OIL

Crush 1 clove of fresh garlic and mix with a tablespoon of olive oil. Let stand for 24–48 hours. Use only the oil; mixture will last up to four days.

HERBAL OILS

Vehicle: Organic olive oil or ghee
Materials: Saucepan; clean cheesecloth strainer; jar for finished compound
Procedure: Mix 1 part dry herb(s) in 16 parts water (i.e., $\frac{1}{2}$ ounce herbs to 8 ounces of water). Simmer slowly over low heat until water is reduced to one-quarter of its original amount (i.e., 2 ounces from the original 8 ounces). Strain. Mix equal amounts of strained herbal liquid with olive oil or ghee (see below). Simmer over low heat until all herbal liquid has evaporated. Oil will remain good for six months. Store at room temperature.

To make ghee: Place 1 pound of organic sweet, unsalted butter in a saucepan. Heat over medium heat until the butter is melted. Turn heat to low and simmer. Stir occasionally with a stainless steel spoon, scraping the bottom. After 10 to 20 minutes, the ghee will turn a golden color and smell a little like popcorn. White curds will form and separate from the clear substance of the ghee. As the whitish curds turn a light brown and the boiling quiets, the ghee is ready. Remove it from the heat and cool to lukewarm. Decant the clear ghee from the curds (which have settled to the bottom) into a clean container and discard the curds. Store ghee covered at room temperature.

HERBAL WINES

Fermentation, the process used in making wine, is an alchemical procedure that releases subtle healing energies from organic substances. Wine made from red grapes works primarily on the Liver/Gallbladder and Heart systems, strengthening their functions and addressing the emotional imbalances that are associated with these systems, such as depression, anxiety, and anger. The Liver and Heart systems control the deeper aspects of the mind-body functions. When wine is mulled (boiled) with herbs, it becomes a strong vehicle for mediating the herb's therapeutic qualities as well as balancing the Liver/Gallbladder and Heart systems.

Vehicle: Organic red wine

Materials: Saucepan; cooking thermometer; clean cheesecloth strainer

Procedure: In a medium saucepan, mix 4 tablespoons of dried herbs and 2 tablespoons organic red wine vinegar with 1 bottle of organic red wine. Simmer slowly for 5 minutes. This will reduce the alcohol to about 2 percent. Let it cool to under 120° Fahrenheit and add $\frac{1}{3}$ cup of organic honey. Heat again for five minutes to just below the boiling point. Skim off foam, strain, and rebottle the wine. Take 1–3 tablespoons daily for up to three weeks.

HERBAL BATHS

Make 1 quart of herbal decoction and add to bath water.

HOMEOPATHICS

The homeopathic process of potentization releases the dynamic life-form energies inherent in all substances. The potentized remedy will bypass the digestive process and be taken up directly into the energy matrix of the body through mucous membranes or skin. Potentized (homeopathic) remedies work more strongly on biological processes than substance-level remedies, such as herbal therapies. All of the spices and herbs mentioned in this book can be made into homeopathic remedies through the procedure outlined below. However, expert knowledge of homeopathic principles is required if working on more advanced levels than indicated in this book.

Vehicle: Distilled water

Materials: One 100-cc beaker graduated in 10-cc increments; one 200-cc glass beaker or test tube with rubber stopper or top; one 30–50 milliliter brown apothecary bottle with dropper (purchase new).

Procedure: Put 1 part of substance or tincture (10 cc) to be potentized in the test tube together with 9 parts (90 cc) of distilled water. Close the end of the test tube with a stopper. Potentize by vigorously shaking up and down for 1 minute, striking the bottom in the hand each time. Pour off 9 parts (90 cc) of the fluid, leaving 1 part (10 cc), and add 9 parts (90 cc) of distilled water. Potentize (shake) again. Repeat this process 1 to 6 times, depending on the degree of potentization desired (each dilution = 1X; diluting (potentizing) five times = 5X).

After final dilution, add $\frac{1}{2}$ teaspoon of pure grain alcohol, such as Everclear or Puro de Cana, to the 30-milliliter brown apothecary bottle and fill with the last potency made. Give 10 drops under the tongue, outside of mealtimes, 1 to 3 times a day, for ten to twenty-four days. Avoid all caffeine while taking the remedy.

FOOD

Spices can be used in preparing foods—add to foods that are lightly boiled or steamed, stir-fried, or raw.

Ailments & Therapies

ACCIDENTS AND TRAUMA

TEACHING

Accidents and traumas pose the greatest immediate challenges to the immune system. Remember that the immune system is an *integration* system that enables us to absorb and deal with the vast number of experiences, stimuli, and substances we come into contact with each day. Though we rarely think of it, our immune system also initiates the stabilizing and healing functions of the body when accidents or traumas have compromised it.

Sometimes an accident or trauma can be so severe that the immune system is required to respond in phases to best stabilize the situation. If you fall and break your arm, for instance, your body and mind begin to integrate all of the aspects of the fall immediately. To do so, many complex mechanisms and systems are activated at the same time: bone tissue metabolism, bone sheath tissue system, connective tissues, nerves, circulation, and lymphatic system, just to name a few. Through the wisdom of the body, these mechanisms simultaneously begin to repair and heal. In order for the body to create a "space" for an immediate, strong, and timely response, it resorts to what we call "shock" to help it begin and accomplish its agenda.

Shock is in reality an important and often lifesaving response of our immune system to overwhelming trauma. Shock affects the whole body and mind. Basically, shock is a partial rerouting of the body's vital energies. The energies required for thinking, moving, and speaking are redirected inward to assist the internal organs with their vital functions. So much energy can be redirected that a person can become unconscious, which is the strongest manifestation of this redirection and compensation process.

Sometimes a person will vomit when confronted with an overwhelming situation. Both vomiting and losing consciousness indicate that the body has

56

closed off certain processes like digesting and thinking. By canceling the functional demands of conscious thinking and the energetic demands of digestion, the body conserves these energies and instead uses them for emergency healing and stabilizing the body's systems. Thus, it is important to eat very lightly after experiencing a trauma. When functioning normally, the body uses about 30 percent of its energies to digest complex foods. During the initial phase of healing after a trauma, the body needs to reroute this energy to the healing process rather than to the digestion of meals.

In all traumas, the body will do a wonderful job in immediately assessing the damage and then creating the best strategy for dealing with it, a strategy that involves redirecting and mobilizing all of its resources in the most efficient and effective way possible. In order to allow a traumatized person's body to do what it knows is best, that person needs three things: *security, calmness, and rest.*

In any trauma, the person involved needs to feel that they are being taken care of and that things will be all right. Fear and worry consume the energies needed in the healing process. Decreasing the person's fear level frees the energies to be used productively. Remember, a traumatized person is not immediately capable of providing himself with calmness and rest; you must create those things for him. Calm him with your presence, regardless of what you know or don't know about the medical aspects of the situation. Your presence, calmness, contact, and reassurance are the most important medicines of the moment. If you are alone with a seriously traumatized or injured person, keep in mind that pain is a sign of the body's working continually to heal itself; that panic and fear will never contribute to any form of healing process, but calmness will; and that the body is so wise as to *always do what is best and most appropriate in any circumstance and under all conditions.*

THERAPY

BURNS

General Recommendations for First-Degree and Second-Degree Burns
Remedy #1
- Lukewarm water

Run lukewarm water on the burn area immediately after being burned. Do this until the pain lessens. Although cold water feels better, lukewarm water hastens the healing, while cold water inhibits the flow of blood and lymph that heal the burn.

Remedy #2

- Aloe vera juice from the plant or commercially prepared gel or juice
- Turmeric powder (if available)

Slice open the leaf from an aloe vera plant and scoop out some of the juice and pulp. With the back of a spoon, mash it into a paste. If you have turmeric powder, put a pinch or two in the paste. Apply the paste to the burn area. Cover with gauze bandages. Repeat as needed.

Remedy #3

- Egg whites

Spread several layers of egg white on the burn area. Let dry without covering. Repeat as needed.

Tissue Salts

For immediate use on first and second degree burns and scalds:

- *Kali mur. 6X*

Take 1 dose internally once an hour up to 6 times. In addition, dissolve 8 tablets in 1 tablespoon of water. Spoon this mixture over the burn and let dry uncovered. Repeat as needed.

After blister forms:

- *Natrum mur. 6X*

Take 1 dose 3 times daily for up to three days while blister is present.

Foods

- **Pineapple**

  THERAPEUTIC ACTION: Promotes healing of burns

  PREPARATION METHOD: Fruit juice compress

  Note: Do not open a blister. It is the major healing mechanism of a burn. Blisters protect layers of connective tissue that, if exposed, become prone to infection. Protect the blister from bursting by covering it with a gauze bandage. After the blister dries, it will peel off revealing the healed skin below.

BLEEDING

For severe bleeding, use first-aid techniques.

Bleeding is the body's response to tissue damage. Blood contains immune substances that repair damaged tissues and cells, as well as nutrients that support the healing and growth of new tissues. Through bleeding, all parts of the wound or lesion come in contact with the life-giving substances of blood.

Bleeding cleanses tissues from the inside out. Any minor wound or lesion should be encouraged to bleed so that you can see the blood coming to the surface before washing the lesion. After you are sure that the blood has been able to do its part in cleansing and bringing its healing materials to all parts of the wound, you can take measures to stop the bleeding. Protect the wound with a gauze bandage until a scab forms. Scabbing is like the blister on a burn—it protects the healing tissues underneath and helps the system complete its work. When you notice a scab itching, it is a sign that the tissues are healing. When the scab becomes completely dry, it will begin to loosen by itself.

General Remedy

- Wet coffee grounds

    Coffee grounds can be applied directly to small wounds to check bleeding.

Tissue Salts

- *Ferrum phos.* 6X

    Take 4 pills every half hour; as bleeding symptoms improve, reduce the frequency of doses.

BRUISES AND SPRAINS

Bruising is the body's way of healing damaged soft tissues located under the skin. When these tissues are damaged, the body rushes blood and lymph to the area. These substances protect, repair, and nourish the tissues. The same holds true of sprains. The swelling that accompanies bruises and sprains is an indication of this increased blood and lymph activity. When we sprain a joint, our ability to move that joint is restricted by pain and swelling. These symptoms are the body's wise way of showing us how to respond: the body is saying, "Don't use me until I've healed!" Pay attention to this wisdom.

You can immediately use a cold pack, such as ice wrapped in a towel. Do not apply the ice directly on the skin. In using cold packs, the idea is to create a strong cooling effect on the skin, but not too cold. Apply the cold pack for 5 minutes, then remove it for 5 minutes. Do this, alternating on and off treatment, up to 10 times. This cycle, which increases circulation in order to promote healing, can be repeated several times a day. Do not use painkillers or ice to stop the healing process and reduce the pain. Even though pain may be significantly reduced, the healing process has been stopped prematurely. Using the compromised joint under these circumstances will cause further damage.

General Remedies

Remedy #1

• Take 1 or 2 of the following: fennel seed powder, cayenne pepper, caraway seed, ginger powder, turmeric powder

Pour 1 cup of boiling water over 1 teaspoon of spice or herb. If using two ingredients, use $\frac{1}{2}$ teaspoon of each ingredient. Let it steep for 10 minutes. Apply liquid to bruise several times a day.

Remedy #2

• Black or green tea bag

Moisten a tea bag with room-temperature water, then place it on the bruise. Leave the tea bag in place for 30 minutes. This can be repeated several times a day.

Remedy #3 (especially good for an eye bruise)

• 1 teaspoon raw potato, peeled and grated
• 1 teaspoon parsley, chopped

Mix together potato and parsley. Wrap mixture in a layer of gauze or piece of clean cotton cloth so that the moisture from the mixture can soak through. Place over the eye or on the bruise for 30 minutes. Repeat 3–5 times per day.

Tissue Salts

• *Ferrum phos.* 6X

Take 3 doses per day for up to three days. If symptoms start to improve, reduce the frequency of doses.

Spices, Herbs, and Foods

• **Cayenne pepper**

THERAPEUTIC ACTION: Promotes healing of bruises, sprains, and wounds; reduces muscle pain and general pain

PREPARATION METHOD: All methods

• **Cardamom**

THERAPEUTIC ACTION: Promotes healing of bruises and sprains

PREPARATION METHOD: All methods

• **Caraway**

THERAPEUTIC ACTION: Promotes healing of bruises; reduces swelling and pain

PREPARATION METHOD: All methods

• **Fennel**

THERAPEUTIC ACTION: Promotes healing of bruises and sprains

PREPARATION METHOD: Standard hot infusion, decoction, herbal compress

- **Potato**
  THERAPEUTIC ACTION: Promotes healing of tendinitis and bruises
  PREPARATION METHOD: Vegetable compress using warm baked pulp of potato
- **Turmeric**
  THERAPEUTIC ACTION: Promotes healing of sprains and strains; acts like cortisone
  PREPARATION METHOD: Standard hot infusion, herbal compress

WOUNDS AND LESIONS

Wounds and lesions need to heal properly. The suggestions listed below will support and speed the healing process.

General Remedies

Remedy #1
- Thyme
- Rosemary
Make a standard hot infusion of either thyme or rosemary or use both together. Wash the wound with the tea several times a day.

Remedy #2
- Aloe vera juice from plant or in gel form
- Turmeric powder (if available)
Slice open the leaf from an aloe vera plant and scoop out some of the juice and pulp. With the back of a spoon, mash it into a paste. If you have turmeric powder, put a pinch or two in the paste. Apply the paste to the wound. Do not cover. Repeat as needed.

Remedy #3
- Lemon juice
- Cane sugar
Mix equal parts lemon juice and cane sugar, then add twice the amount of water. Wash wound several times a day with mixture.

Remedy #4
- Honey
Place honey directly on wound.

Remedy #5
- Cayenne pepper
- Olive oil or ghee
Prepare herbal oil with above ingredients (see Remedy Preparation Tech-

niques). Apply oil directly to wound. If oil is not available, apply powdered cayenne directly on the wound.

Spices, Herbs, and Foods

- **Onions/leeks**
  THERAPEUTIC ACTION: Promotes healing of wounds
  PREPARATION METHOD: Herbal compress
- **Rosemary**
  THERAPEUTIC ACTION: Promotes healing of wounds, insect bites, and stings
  PREPARATION METHOD: All methods
- **Thyme**
  THERAPEUTIC ACTION: Promotes healing of wounds; repels insects
  PREPARATION METHOD: Standard hot infusion, decoction, herbal compress

BEE AND WASP STINGS AND INSECT BITES

Some insects, such as bees, wasps, and spiders, use a venom for protection or to hunt for food. These substances are a natural and necessary part of the insect's life. If you are bitten or stung by one of these insects, its venom will tend to produce a reaction. For most people, these reactions are mildly unpleasant and abate within a few hours. However, some people, because of functional issues in their immune system, are highly allergic to insect bites. If you have problems of this nature, apply one of the suggestions below and call emergency medical service immediately. But remain calm, as worrying will not help. Your body is working to resolve the issue in the most efficient and effective way possible.

General Remedies

Remedy #1
- $\frac{1}{2}$ teaspoon sugar
- $\frac{1}{2}$ teaspoon cinnamon
- $\frac{1}{2}$ teaspoon anise seed powder
- water

Mix together the sugar, cinnamon, and anise seed powder. If only sugar is available, just use that ingredient. Add enough water to make a paste. Apply mixture directly to the sting and the surrounding area.

Remedy #2
- 1 clove garlic
- $\frac{1}{2}$ teaspoon salt

Crush the garlic and mix with the salt. Apply directly to sting.

Remedy #3

- Black or green tea bag

Moisten the tea bag in room-temperature water and apply directly to bite.

Remedy #4

- Apple cider vinegar

Soak a clean cloth with the vinegar and place on the sting.

Tissue Salts

- *Natrum mur.* 6X

Take 1 dose 4 times a day, for up to three days, reducing the number of dosages per day as symptoms improve.

Homeopathy

- *Apis mellifica* 200C

If you are allergic to bee stings, purchase this remedy from a health food store. Take 1 dose immediately after being stung. You can repeat the dose, only once more, after 20 minutes,. If you are hyperallergic to bee stings, seek medical help immediately.

Spices, Herbs, and Foods

- **Anise seed**

  THERAPEUTIC ACTION: Promotes healing of animal and insect bites; is an antidote to poisons

  PREPARATION METHOD: Herbal compress

- **Basil**

  THERAPEUTIC ACTION: Promotes healing of insect and animal bites, is an antidote to poisons, repels insects

  PREPARATION METHOD: Standard hot infusion, fresh plant tincture, dry plant tincture, herbal compress

- **Black pepper**

  THERAPEUTIC ACTION: Promotes healing of animal bites

  PREPARATION METHOD: Standard hot infusion, dry plant tincture, herbal compress

- **Cardamom**

  THERAPEUTIC ACTION: Promotes healing of bruises, sprains, and insect stings

  PREPARATION METHOD: All methods

- **Cinnamon**

  THERAPEUTIC ACTION: Promotes healing of animal and insect bites; repels insects

PREPARATION METHOD: Standard hot infusion, herbal compress

- **Rosemary**

  THERAPEUTIC ACTION: Promotes healing of wounds, insect bites, and stings

  PREPARATION METHOD: All methods

POISON IVY AND POISON OAK

Plants such as poison ivy and poison oak have plant toxins on the surface of their leaves or stems. These toxins are part of the plant's metabolic system and prevent certain plant predators from attacking them. Our skin temporarily reacts to these substances. The suggestions below will help reduce the symptoms and return the skin to its normal state.

General Remedies

Remedy #1

- 1 fresh, raw cucumber

  Finely chop a cucumber using a blender or slice thinly. Apply directly to skin and hold in place with a cloth. Repeat as needed.

Remedy #2

- $\frac{1}{2}$ cup baking soda

  Add baking soda to a cool bath and soak.

Tissue Salts

- *Kali sulph.* 6X

  Take 1 dose per hour up to 6 times on the first day; 1 dose up to 4 times the next day; 1 dose 3 times on the following day; reduce the number of dosages per day as soon as symptoms begin to improve.

SUNBURN

Sunburn is something that can be avoided by being prudent while in the sun. When exposing parts of the body directly to the sun, such as while swimming, do not wait until you feel the skin starting to react, but seek shade and cover the body with a light layer of clothing. After exposure to the sun, it is a good idea to rub some organic olive oil on the skin. This will reduce the effect of the drying and heating energies of the sun.

General Remedies

Remedy #1

- 3 tablespoons of oatmeal

- $\frac{1}{2}$ cup of water

Mix the oatmeal and water and bring to a boil. Simmer for 6 minutes. Let the mixture cool. Wrap in gauze and apply to burn.

Or wrap $\frac{1}{2}$ cup dry oatmeal in cheesecloth and steep 15 minutes in 3 cups of boiling water. Remove oatmeal sac from the water. Apply liquid when cool directly to the burn. Repeat application several times.

Remedy #2
- 1 quart of water
- Three tea bags each of one or more of the following types of tea: peppermint, chamomile, and lemon

Bring the water to a boil in a nonaluminum pot. Add tea bags and steep for 20 minutes. Pour entire standard hot infusion into a bath. Soak in bathwater for at least 10 minutes.

Note: The juice of one lemon can be used instead of lemon tea.

Remedy #3
- Apple cider vinegar

Apply the vinegar directly to the sunburn.

AGING: CARE OF THE ELDERLY

TEACHING

Our society tends to view aging as a negative process, one that threatens life's quality and the body's health. Menopause, for instance, is often treated like a disease, as though nature built in a self-destruct mechanism for anyone over the age of fifty. Moreover, the elderly are often seen as nonproductive individuals who no longer contribute to the mainstream of society and have become mere spectators of life, consuming medical care and whatever time and attention others can spare. Many elderly individuals passively await the end of their life.

This attitude not only causes but also promotes the very thing we fear—the loss of self-worth. Such a loss is communal as well as personal: by excluding the elderly from the active agendas of our communities, we lose the wisdom, experience, and knowledge that reside within many of our older citizens. We need to shift our viewpoint and consider the natural last stage of life as the crowning of our personal maturation and evolution, the point at which our lives have ripened into the fullness of meaning and greater consciousness.

The Three Major Periods of Life

Traditional health and medical systems view the elderly's physical abilities, general health, and role in society quite differently. To understand this viewpoint, it helps to consider the three major periods of development and maturation that occur throughout the life of a human being:

- The first stage of development extends from birth to puberty.

- The second stage spans puberty to about age fifty.

- The final stage begins at fifty and covers the remainder of life.

Each stage unfolds its inherent gifts and challenges to further our development and make us more creative and fulfilled persons. In addition, each stage offers a sacred worthiness that brings growth and meaning to our lives and the lives of those around us. We need to recognize that each period of our life contributes something essential and inspiring to our personal evolution and thereby assists us in reaching our full potential.

During each life stage, our physical functions and our consciousness develop inversely. As consciousness expands through the experiences encountered in daily living, the physical body's vitality diminishes. Observe a one-year-old child: his intellectual abilities are relatively undeveloped due to the fact that his experience is very limited, but the bodily functions at this stage are extremely strong and supple. When injured, the body heals quickly and physical growth proceeds at a rapid pace. In comparison, an elderly person has the expanded consciousness resulting from years of experience, but his bodily functions are less vital and the body is less supple. The wisdom of consciousness produced during the life process is observably much greater than that of the one-year-old, in whom consciousness is more dedicated to the body's growth and its sensory processes. Notice how the physical body "feeds" the consciousness from its own vitality; and as the consciousness expands through experience, the body's vitality lessens. We experience this phenomenon when we become tired from periods of concentrated thinking and using our mental faculties.

After the age of fifty, our biological energies change from a higher to a lower level of metabolism. Energies usually directed to outer activities—such as career building, forming a home and family, and building tissues to support such activities—turn inward to complete our maturation. During this last stage of development, all aspects of our person become more visible. Our attitudes, behavior, and health mirror everything that has happened in our life. If we fostered love and understanding as best we could, we will become even more loving and understanding with age. If we allowed ourselves to become bitter or fearful in the building phase of our lives, we will become the images of bitterness or fearfulness in our final maturing process. We must remember that the world does not create us, we create the world. We become what we create in our heart, the center of our personhood.

Health in the Final Stage of Maturity

As these energies of maturation and their new patterns settle into the body, unresolved health issues become more systemic and begin to manifest themselves more strongly, just as emotional issues do. Symptoms like arthritis and heart disease, for example, are due more to poor lifestyle habits and not maintaining the body's health while younger than to old age. This manifestation of symptoms promotes the idea that elderly people are "sickly" and that the aging process is responsible. In the strictest sense, this assumption is incorrect: aging is not a disease, nor does it produce disease. However, just as the maturation process reveals more about us, it also reveals more about how we have dealt with our health in the past. Health issues that have not been corrected have also "matured" and manifest themselves more openly.

It is important that the elderly receive the care they need in order to maintain their health and preserve their life quality. Unfortunately, the elderly have become one of the main targets of the medical industry. Statistics show that, on average, every American over the age of fifty is on at least two daily long-term prescription drugs. In some cases, a person's health may have deteriorated to such an extent that he or she can only live through the chemical intervention afforded by drugs. Chemical drugs may be necessary because the person previously has been unable to receive proper health care or earlier treatments have not resolved her health issues. Often, simple natural therapies will deal with health issues, without the serious side effects of drugs.

THERAPY

To Support Cell Nutrition

Tissue Salts

- *Silicea 6X*

  Take 1 dose per day for two weeks, then a pause for three weeks. Repeat cycle as needed.

INSOMNIA IN THE ELDERLY

Tissue Salts

- *Kali phos.* 6X
- *Natrum phos.* 6X
- *Natrum mur.* 6X

  Take 1 dose of each together before bedtime.

Reflexology

For instructions on reflexology, see "Reflexology" under "How to Use the Therapy Section" at the beginning of Part II.

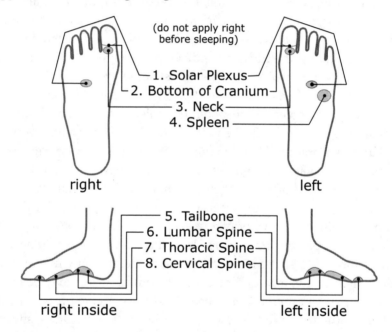

right

left

right inside

left inside

CONSTIPATION IN THE ELDERLY

Tissue Salts

- *Kali mur.* 6X
- *Natrum phos.* 6X
- *Ferrum phos.* 6X
- *Calc. phos.* 6X

  These remedies can be taken together. Take 1 dose of each up to 3 times daily for one week. Reduce dosage as symptoms begin to improve.

Reflexology

For instructions on reflexology, see "Reflexology" under "How to Use the Therapy Section" at the beginning of Part II.

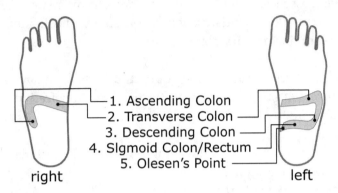

1. Ascending Colon
2. Transverse Colon
3. Descending Colon
4. Sigmoid Colon/Rectum
5. Olesen's Point

right   left

CONVALESCENCE AFTER AN ILLNESS

- *Calc. phos.* 6X

Take 1 dose up to 3 times daily for one week. Reduce the number of dosages per day as symptoms begin improving.

(For additional therapy suggestions for specific health problems, see the appropriate sections.)

GENERAL CARE OF THE ELDERLY

Spices and Herbs

- **Basil**

THERAPEUTIC ACTION: Lifts the spirit; restores brain functions and thinking processes; restores strength

PREPARATION METHOD: Standard hot infusion, standard cold infusion, decoction, fresh plant tincture, dry plant tincture

- **Black pepper**

THERAPEUTIC ACTION: Relieves all deficient conditions

PREPARATION METHOD: Dry plant tincture; include in the daily diet

- **Cayenne pepper**

THERAPEUTIC ACTION: Stimulates all vital processes; increases circulation; reduces weakness, fatigue, and slow responses; increases vital heat

PREPARATION METHOD: Dry plant tincture; include in the daily diet

- **Chicory**

THERAPEUTIC ACTION: Decreases debility; helps with poor vision; strengthens the body after chronic illness; alleviates poor digestion; restores blood; increases vital essence; strengthens nerves; prevents premature aging

PREPARATION METHOD: Standard hot infusion, standard cold infusion, decoction, fresh plant tincture, dry plant tincture

- **Ginger**

THERAPEUTIC ACTION: General tonic; supports digestion; enhances circulation

PREPARATION METHOD: Standard hot infusion, decoction, fresh plant tincture, dry plant tincture

- **Green tea**

THERAPEUTIC ACTION: Retards the aging process; mild stimulant; enhances and strengthens the immune system

PREPARATION METHOD: Standard hot infusion

- **Marjoram**

THERAPEUTIC ACTION: General tonic

PREPARATION METHOD: Standard hot infusion, decoction, dry plant tincture

- **Parsley**

THERAPEUTIC ACTION: Restorative tonic

PREPARATION METHOD: Standard hot infusion, standard cold infusion, decoction, fresh plant tincture, herbal wine

- **Sage**

THERAPEUTIC ACTION: Reduces mental exhaustion; enhances concentration; aids depression

PREPARATION METHOD: Standard hot infusion, decoction, fresh plant tincture, dry plant tincture (For depression, add $\frac{1}{4}$ teaspoon of crushed cloves.)

Foods

- **Almonds**

THERAPEUTIC ACTION: Stimulates brain functions; improves memory; softens bowels and aids digestion

PREPARATION METHOD: Dry plant tincture; include in the daily diet. Dip almonds in sugar water made from cane sugar; eat 4–6 almonds twice daily.

- **Apricot**

THERAPEUTIC ACTION: Restorative tonic

PREPARATION METHOD: Include in the daily diet

- **Artichoke**

THERAPEUTIC ACTION: Retards the aging process; builds cells; restores vital essence; strengthens nerves

PREPARATION METHOD: Include in the daily diet 2–3 times per week

- **Asparagus**

THERAPEUTIC ACTION: Nourishes and replenishes deficient systems; restores blood; increases vital essence; brightens vision; strengthens sinews; reduces senility; helps with brittle bones; helps blurred vision; eases debility; relieves joint and muscle pains; helps chronic bladder irritation

PREPARATION METHOD: Include in the diet 2–3 times per week

- **Barley**

THERAPEUTIC ACTION: Very nutritious; calming and strengthening effect on the heart and circulation; reduces cholesterol; antitumor, antiviral properties

PREPARATION METHOD: Include in the diet

- **Beets**

THERAPEUTIC ACTION: General tonic; replenishes blood; supports tissue immunity

PREPARATION METHOD: Include in the diet

- **Carrots**

THERAPEUTIC ACTION: Decreases debility; increases strength during convalescence; a good tonic; cleanses the bowels

PREPARATION METHOD: Include in the diet 3–5 times per week

- **Chickpeas**

THERAPEUTIC ACTION: Supports convalescence; strengthens weakened nerves

PREPARATION METHOD: Include in the diet

- **Dried figs or prunes**

THERAPEUTIC ACTION: Improves constipation; promotes healthy bowels

PREPARATION METHOD: Dried fruit technique (prepare with a pinch of anise)

- **Egg shells**

THERAPEUTIC ACTION: Builds bone tissue; helps resolve osteoporosis and brittle bones

PREPARATION METHOD: Wash egg shells from organic eggs in cold water. Let them dry completely, then crush the shells with a pestle or rolling pin to a powder. Sprinkle one teaspoon of powder on any food once a day.

- **Fenugreek and flaxseeds**

THERAPEUTIC ACTION: Aids digestion; cleanses bowels and digestive tract

PREPARATION METHOD: Crush 1 teaspoon of fenugreek seeds and 1 teaspoon of flaxseeds. Add 1 cup of boiling water and steep for 8 minutes. Add a pinch of ginger powder. Drink with the seeds.

- **Pure raw cane sugar**

THERAPEUTIC ACTION: Strengthens weakened nerves; reduces anemia

PREPARATION METHOD: Include 1 teaspoon in the daily diet

• **Salmon bones**

THERAPEUTIC ACTION: Builds bone tissue; helps resolve osteoporosis and brittle bones

PREPARATION METHOD: Wash the large vertebra bones from a salmon in cold water. Let dry completely, then crush with a pestle or with rolling pin to a powder. Sprinkle 1 teaspoon of powder on any food once a day.

Reflexology

For instructions on reflexology, see "Reflexology" under "How to Use the Therapy Section" at the beginning of Part II.

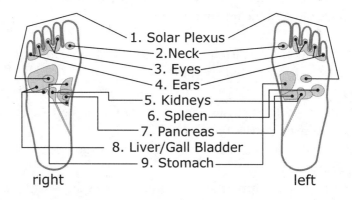

1. Solar Plexus
2. Neck
3. Eyes
4. Ears
5. Kidneys
6. Spleen
7. Pancreas
8. Liver/Gall Bladder
9. Stomach

right   left

CLEANSING THE BODY

TEACHING

One of the ways that the body works to ensure its continued health is by eliminating toxins from its systems, tissues, and cells. A toxin is a substance that is foreign to the body and inhibits or damages its functions or a substance that the body cannot metabolize or use to nourish itself.

There are three major sources of toxins. One is the chemicals and substances with which we come into contact in our immediate environment. These include the chemicals in household items and industrial pollution; chemicals in prescription and nonprescription drugs, dental materials, and vaccines; and the chemical additives, including insecticides, pesticides, and fertilizers in our food and water.

The second source is the toxins that the body produces through incomplete or poor metabolism of what it ingests. These toxins result from poor digestion, constipation, shallow breathing, and lack of exercise. We must also remember that the mind produces toxins that affect the body. Fear, anger, and insecurity, for instance, affect the body's biochemistry, resulting in toxins that affect tissues and cells and need to be detoxified by the body's systems.

The third source is the toxins that occur from activities in the immune system. Healing processes in the body's tissues usually involve microbes. The metabolic products of microbes, as well as the antigens they contain that help to stimulate the immune system, are in the long run toxic to the body. When the immune system is resolving microbial issues as part of the healing process, the body needs to detoxify itself. If the original cause of the health issue is not completely resolved due to functional disturbances in systems that influence the immune system, the problem becomes chronic. Furthermore, the immune system becomes exhausted through its constant elevated response and the buildup of toxins, even if the original symptoms improve. Exhaustion of the immune system is present in all chronic health issues. We must remember that symptoms indicate that the immune system is doing its job. When the symptoms disappear, either the immune processes have resolved the issue or the immune system has become exhausted and is no longer able to sustain its work, allowing the original issue to change its patterns and move deeper, spreading through the body's systems, and manifesting itself in other ways. This mechanism is the basis of what we call "chronic disease."

THERAPY

TOXIN AND PARASITE CLEANSE

General Remedies

Remedy #1
- 1 teaspoon apple cider vinegar (preferably organic)
- $\frac{1}{3}$ cup water

Mix vinegar with water. Drink in sips 1–2 times daily. *Do not use when there are symptoms of indigestion, such as loose stools.* Apple cider vinegar removes toxins and parasites from the body, as well as the after-effects of food poisoning.

Remedy #2
- 1 rounded teaspoon of dried basil or 2 teaspoons crushed fresh basil
- $\frac{1}{4}$ teaspoon powdered cloves

Prepare a standard hot infusion using either fresh or dried basil. Add powdered cloves. Drink once daily for ten days.

DISEASE TOXIN CLEANSE REMEDY

General Remedies

- 1 large onion
- 3 garlic cloves
- 2 quarts of water

Chop onion into $\frac{1}{2}$-inch cubes and slice three peeled garlic cloves. Place garlic and onions in a bowl and add water. Place the bowl in the sun from 10 A.M. to 2 P.M. Strain and refrigerate liquid. Drink 2 ounces (1 shot glass) once daily for a week. Repeat as necessary.

CLEANSING THE INTESTINAL SYSTEM; PROMOTING BOWEL FUNCTION

General Remedies

Remedy #1
- 1 teaspoon flaxseeds
- 1 teaspoon fenugreek seeds
- 1 cup boiling water

Grind fenugreek and fresh flaxseeds separately (grind to a granule). Mix them together and pour boiling water over the mixture. Let it steep for 8 minutes. Drink liquid, including the seeds, once per day for a week. Repeat cycle as necessary.

Remedy #2
- Juice of $\frac{1}{2}$ lemon
- 1 teaspoon fresh castor or olive oil
- 1 pinch ginger powder

Mix the lemon juice in water. Add teaspoon olive oil or castor oil and a pinch of ginger powder. Drink 1 cup daily for two weeks. Pause for two weeks, then repeat the cycle.

GENERAL CLEANSING OF THE BODY

Spices and Herbs

- **Chicory**
  THERAPEUTIC ACTION: Promotes cleansing, clears toxins
  PREPARATION METHOD: Include in the diet
- **Fennel**
  THERAPEUTIC ACTION: Internal cleansing
  PREPARATION METHOD: Standard hot infusion (crush seeds), decoction; include in the diet

- **Fenugreek**
  THERAPEUTIC ACTION: Internal cleansing
  PREPARATION METHOD: Include in the diet
- **Garlic**
  THERAPEUTIC ACTION: Clears toxins and parasites; antidotes poisons
  PREPARATION METHOD: Include in the diet
- **Ginger**
  THERAPEUTIC ACTION: Internal cleansing
  PREPARATION METHOD: Standard hot infusion; include in the diet
- **Parsley**
  THERAPEUTIC ACTION: Internal cleansing
  PREPARATION METHOD: Decoction, fresh plant tincture; include in the diet
- **Sage**
  THERAPEUTIC ACTION: Internal cleansing
  PREPARATION METHOD: Standard hot infusion, fresh plant tincture, dry plant tincture; include in the diet

Foods

- **Apple**
  THERAPEUTIC ACTION: Internal cleansing
  PREPARATION METHOD: Include in the diet
- **Artichoke**
  THERAPEUTIC ACTION: Cleanses the body internally; stimulates liver functions
  PREPARATION METHOD: Include in the diet
- **Asparagus**
  THERAPEUTIC ACTION: Promotes cleansing; clears toxins
  PREPARATION METHOD: Include in the diet
- **Beets**
  THERAPEUTIC ACTION: Internal cleansing
  PREPARATION METHOD: Include in the diet
- **Carrot juice (with pulp)**
  THERAPEUTIC ACTION: Internal cleansing
  PREPARATION METHOD: Drink with a pinch of ginger powder added
- **Celery**
  THERAPEUTIC ACTION: Internal cleansing; clears toxins; cleans kidneys and liver
  PREPARATION METHODS: Decoction, fresh plant tincture; include in the diet
- **Onions**
  THERAPEUTIC ACTION: Internal cleansing
  PREPARATION METHOD: Include in the diet

- **Potato and celery**

  THERAPEUTIC ACTION: Internal cleansing

  PREPARATION METHOD: Include in the diet

- **Turnips**

  THERAPEUTIC ACTION: Internal cleansing

  PREPARATION METHOD: Include in the diet

Reflexology

For instructions on reflexology, see "Reflexology" under "How to Use the Therapy Section" at the beginning of Part II.

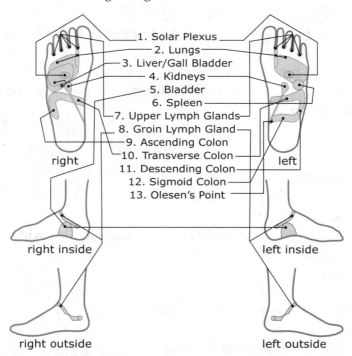

1. Solar Plexus
2. Lungs
3. Liver/Gall Bladder
4. Kidneys
5. Bladder
6. Spleen
7. Upper Lymph Glands
8. Groin Lymph Gland
9. Ascending Colon
10. Transverse Colon
11. Descending Colon
12. Sigmoid Colon
13. Olesen's Point

right

left

right inside

left inside

right outside

left outside

COLDS AND FLU

TEACHING

A cold enables the body to readjust itself to stress factors. When the body has to deal with strong stimuli like excessive cold, heat, drafts, dampness, or exhausting activities, it may become stressed. Situations such as moving, meeting a deadline, or losing a loved one can also create stress. A common cold is not a disease, but a response from the immune system that cleanses the body of the reactions to stress and, in so doing, strengthens the immune system itself.

Microbes and Health

Conventional medicine often blames microbes for causing colds. Many people don't know that not all scientists agree with this belief. In fact, most practitioners of Classical medicine take the stance that microbes do not cause colds and only appear *after* the first symptoms have manifested. Microbes are often present in immune responses as helpers that assist the immune system. In treating colds, we don't want to fight microbes. Rather, we want to do things that support the immune system so that it can accomplish what it needs to do.

We often use the word *flu* when we really mean "cold." True influenza is a viral manifestation, not a bacterial one. Often antibiotics are used to treat flu because colds and influenza share many of the same symptoms. Antibiotics, of course, have no effect on virus activity.

The three major groups of microbes—bacteria, viruses, and yeast—each relate to a specific embryological tissue system and only occur in issues that are produced by that particular tissue system. In the healing activity of the immune system, bacteria and mycobacteria (yeasts) are associated with the nutritive aspect of the body's cells as well as the organs of the digestive tract that are produced by the endoderm embryological system, which includes the stomach, liver, intestines, and the connective tissue. Sinus, throat, and lung "infections" can contain bacterial activity and, though these organs are not usually thought of as being digestive in nature, they do belong to the extended digestive system. Wherever there are cells connected to organs with mucous membranes, there can be bacterial activity.

Viruses are associated with the central nervous system and the brain, both of which are produced by the ectoderm embryological system. All tissues have cells that receive nerve signals from the body's nerve system. Viruses respond to the healing activity in these types of cells whether they are in mucous membrane tissues, connective tissues, or nerve tissues. Stress and conflicts that weaken the nerve system can trigger viral activity. Often, the stresses that overstimulate our nerve system originate in our environment. Most true influenzas, for instance, occur in crowded conditions like big cities, in more extreme stress conditions like war or natural disasters, or in the personal conflicts and stresses that can occur in our school or work environments.

It is important to remember that bacteria and viruses become problems *only* when the immune system has been weakened by common factors in our daily life and is unable to resolve the healing process in a timely manner. That is why maintaining a lifestyle with proper diet and exercise and avoiding harmful toxins in our food and environment are so important for good health.

Microbes don't *cause* disease—we become diseased by having the functions of our body weakened by stress, toxins, chronic ill health, or unhealthy lifestyles. For example, if ten people work in an office where an outbreak of flu occurs, not more than half of them will get the flu even though they were all exposed to it. The half that *doesn't* get the flu is healthy enough that their immune systems are not only able to deal with exposure to the virus, but at the same time, have been able to integrate the stresses encountered in daily life. When stressors from our immediate territory like work, home, and school become too severe or last too long, they harm and exhaust the body, causing the immune system to respond. This response can include virus activity as part of the deeper healing process.

Allergies

Allergy symptoms are often confused with cold and flu symptoms. As with colds and flu, the symptoms of allergies are primary responses of the immune system and its activity in the mucous membranes, and frequently involve the eyes, upper respiratory tract, skin, and digestive tract. During an allergic reaction, the immune system demonstrates that it is still strong and vital, but it also shows that it is reacting in the wrong place at the wrong time and for the wrong reasons. Most allergic reactions occur from contact with natural substances like pollen, dust, mites, and some foods. We should not be reacting at all to these things, which are found normally in nature and do not in any way pose a threat to our health. Allergic reactions clearly indicate that our immune system is compromised because it is reacting to harmless natural substances as though the body needed to heal itself from contact with them. Substances that cause allergic reactions are called allergens. Allergens are not the cause of the immune system being out of balance and reacting improperly. Some other factor (or set of factors) has compromised the immune system and its normal way of responding. These factors are the true cause of allergies. The main culprits are the toxins found in foods, medicines, vaccines, dental amalgam fillings, and root canals, as well as chronic stress and factors that compromise the reproductive organs, such as the use of IUDs and birth control pills. All of these damage the immune system and cause it to react to otherwise harmless substances.

The Healing Process

The inflammation brought on by colds and flu help the immune system cleanse the body's tissues and destroy unneeded microbes and other biological substances like toxins:

- Mucous membranes clean out toxins by forming mucus.

- Fever increases metabolism as part of the healing process.

- Swelling transports new blood and immune substances to areas in need.

- The aches and pains of colds and flu are signs of increased activity and indicate that the body is working to heal itself.

Inflammation and infections only pose a problem when one does not take proper care of them. Suggestions in this chapter will show you how to support the immune system in the healing process.

Our bodies know how to heal—they're created that way. By using natural, often simple therapies, you are not only helping the immune system to complete its work supporting the body's own healing functions, but you are also dealing with the *causes* that produced the inflammation or infection in the first place. We need not fear colds and flu. We have only to listen to what the body tells us through its own body language, which is the language of symptoms, and then respond with confidence. The body is on our side and will do everything in its power to heal itself.

Everyone experiences inflammation of mucous membranes at one time or another; it is a sign of a healthy body. From infancy to the age of puberty, the mucous membranes are very active. Children often experience more periods of inflammation than do adults. Such increased inflammation is due to the maturing processes of body and mind, processes that are connected to the deeper integrating work of the immune system. Inflammation helps the body adjust to its new life and environment, both emotionally and physically. Other factors that can cause chronic (repeated) inflammations are the use of antibiotics (which kill bacteria but don't address causes), allergies, vaccines (which affect the immune system functions and tissues), toxins released by mercury fillings, allergies, and toxins from chemicals in our food and environment.

THERAPY

The immune system works in stages; each stage represents a step in the way that the body is healing itself. The body is a magnificent organism and tells us, if we observe carefully, how and what it's doing to achieve health and balance. Different stages of the immune process produce different symptoms.

Each symptom reveals a picture of what's happening in the body and teaches us how best to respond with a treatment.

The quality of the mucus coming from the nose or throat, for example, tells us much about what is going on in the body. In the first stage of an inflammation, the mucus discharged from the mucous membranes is clear and watery. It can sometimes sting and irritate the skin when in contact with it. In the second stage, the mucus is whitish and usually thicker than in the first stage. In the third stage, the mucus will be yellowish or greenish and can be mixed with a little blood. This type of mucus is filled with cells from the immune system and with microbes that the body no longer needs and has destroyed. The blood, if present, shows us that the body is cleansing itself and rebuilding the mucous membranes that have been working hard to protect and heal the body. The blood comes from the very small blood vessels that bring nutrients and immune substances to the mucous membranes.

Remember, especially if you have small children, that the *first* indications of an immune response, no matter where or why, are changes of normal behavior. Loss of appetite or being fussy with food, unusual irritability, restlessness, excessive tiredness, and dissatisfaction with things or play that usually satisfy are all signs of an active immune response. This is the time to respond by giving rest, cutting down on foods, observing carefully, and being patient.

Remember that one of the best remedies for all symptoms is *rest*.

STAGES OF INFLAMMATION

Tissue Salts

First Stage of Colds and Flu:

Symptoms may include a stronger fever, flushed skin, overall soreness or achiness, a runny nose with clear, often stinging mucus, a reddened or sore throat, a psychological feeling of tiredness, lack of enthusiasm, lack of energy, or restlessness.

- *Ferrum phos.* 6X
- *Mag. phos.* 6X

Take these two remedies together. (See Third Stage of Colds and Flu for doasge.)

Second Stage of Colds and Flu:

After the cold has begun to settle in, the symptoms may include swollen glands, a pale or whitish tongue, a stuffed-up sensation, possibly grey or whitish color in the throat, intermittent fever, chills, lack of appetite, and feelings of discouragement or discontentment. If mucus is present, it will be whitish and thicker.

- *Kali mur.* 6X
- *Silicea* 6X

Take these two remedies together. (See Third Stage of Colds and Flu for doasge.)

Third Stage of Colds and Flu:

In this last stage of inflammation, any mucus will be yellowish or greenish. The tongue will have a tendency to be yellowish, the tonsils may be swollen, and fever usually will rise in the evening and lower somewhat in the morning. Psychologically, you may be irritable, fret over trifles, and feel disheartened.

- *Kali sulph.* 6X
- *Natrum sulph.* 6X
- *Silicea* 6X

Take these three remedies together.

On the first day, take 1 dose every ½ hour *until there is any change in the symptoms.* When *any* of the original symptoms *improve,* reduce the dosage to every 2 hours, but not for more than one day. Then take 3 times daily for three additional days. If symptoms *change,* for example, from the first stage of inflammation, with clear mucus, higher fever, and sharp pains to the second stage, more stuffiness and whitish mucus, then start using the remedies that match the symptoms as explained above. For adults, one dose equals 4 tablets. For children under ten, one dose is 2 tablets.

Foods

- When fever is present, eat only *small* amounts of food containing vital nutrition, such as vegetable broths and foods that are lightly cooked, steamed, or stir-fried. *Only eat foods when there is a natural appetite for them.*

- Drink plenty of water.

- Avoid caffeine, processed sugars, dairy products, wheat products, and foods containing additives, preservatives, MSG, food dyes, artificial flavors, eggs, peanuts, soy products, meats, corn oil, safflower oil, and sunflower oil.

    Use the following foods:
    Olive oil (in stir-frying)
    Carrot juice or grated carrot with every meal, if possible
    Parsley (raw or lightly boiled) with every meal, if possible
    Avocado

Green pepper (cooked, baked, or stir-fried)
Broccoli (lightly cooked)
Cabbage (lightly boiled)
Kale (steamed, medium boiled, or stir-fried)
Onions (boiled, stir-fried, or baked)
Spinach (lightly cooked or stir-fried)
Potato (mashed)
Rice (boiled well)
Apple (grated or juice)
Cranberries (medium cooked or juice)
Red grapes (juice)
Honey
Orange juice
Pineapple juice
Raw cane sugar (only a little)

COLD OR FLU WITH HEADACHE OR UPSET STOMACH

General Remedies

Remedy #1

• 1 teaspoon dried or 1 tablespoon fresh, oregano, thyme, hyssop or chamomile, crushed

• 1 cup of hot water

• 1 tablespoon lemon juice (optional)

• Honey (optional)

Make a tea by steeping 1 teaspoon of dried herb or 1 tablespoon of fresh herb in hot water for 6–7 minutes. If readily available, add lemon juice and sweeten with honey. Take 3 cups per day.

Remedy #2

• $\frac{1}{2}$ teaspoon fennel seed, crushed

• $\frac{1}{2}$ teaspoon coriander powder

• $\frac{1}{2}$ teaspoon peppermint leaf, crushed

• $\frac{1}{8}$ teaspoon ginger powder

• $\frac{1}{2}$ teaspoon marjoram

• $\frac{1}{2}$ teaspoon thyme

To prepare an herbal inhalant, mix ingredients in a bowl. Pour 1 quart of boiling water over mixture. Inhale steam. You can place a towel over your head and let the towel also drape around the bowl.

Mucus Coming from the Sinuses or Being Coughed Up

General Remedies

Remedy #1

- 1 teaspoon of dried or 1 tablespoon fresh, oregano, thyme, hyssop, or chamomile, crushed
- 1 tablespoon lemon juice (opt.)
- Honey (opt.)

Make a tea by steeping 1 teaspoon of dried herb or 1 tablespoon of fresh herb in 1 cup of hot water for 6–7 minutes. If readily available, add 1 tablespoon of lemon juice and sweeten with honey. Take 3 cups per day.

Remedy #2—Inhalant Tea

- $\frac{1}{2}$ teaspoon fennel seed, crushed
- $\frac{1}{2}$ teaspoon coriander powder
- $\frac{1}{2}$ teaspoon peppermint leaf, crushed
- $\frac{1}{8}$ teaspoon ginger powder
- $\frac{1}{2}$ teaspoon marjoram
- $\frac{1}{2}$ teaspoon thyme
- 1 quart of boiling water

To prepare an herbal inhalant, mix herbs and spices in a bowl. Pour boiling water over mixture. Inhale steam. You can place a towel over your head and let the towel also drape around the bowl.

Remedy #3

- $\frac{1}{2}$ cup of water
- $\frac{1}{2}$ teaspoon salt

If there is mucus in the nose, prepare nose drops. Boil the water. Let it cool to lukewarm. Dissolve the salt in the water. Lie down and tilt the head back. Using an eye dropper, place 5 drops of the saltwater into each nostril and let the drops flow back deep into the nose. Wait about 1 minute before sitting upright.

Remedy #4

- Juice of $\frac{1}{2}$ of a lemon
- 8 ounces of water

Drink the lemon juice in water twice daily.

Remedy #5

- 1 teaspoon salt
- 1 cup of warm water
- A few pinches of turmeric powder (if available)

To reduce inflammation and swelling and soothe a sore throat, dissolve salt in warm water. Add turmeric. Gargle. Repeat every 3 hours.

Tissue Salts

See Stages of Inflammation on page 80.

GENERAL CARE OF COLDS AND FLU

Spices and Herbs

- **Basil**

THERAPEUTIC ACTION: Restrains infections; enhances immune system; reduces fever

PREPARATION METHOD: Standard hot infusion, decoction, fresh plant tincture, dry plant tincture

- **Cayenne pepper**

THERAPEUTIC ACTION: Enhances immunity during first stage of colds or flu; antibacterial, antiviral

PREPARATION METHOD: Use to season food

- **Chicory**

THERAPEUTIC ACTION: Reduces fevers

PREPARATION METHOD: Standard hot infusion, fresh plant tincture

- **Cinnamon**

THERAPEUTIC ACTION: Enhances immunity during first stage of colds or flu; antibacterial, antiviral

PREPARATION METHOD: Decoction (using cinnamon sticks/bark), dry plant tincture

- **Cloves**

THERAPEUTIC ACTION: Anti-inflammatory; antibacterial; antiviral

PREPARATION METHOD: Standard hot infusion, dry plant tincture, herbal wine

- **Fennel seed**

THERAPEUTIC ACTION: Preventative for influenza; anti-inflammatory, reduces fever

PREPARATION METHOD: Standard hot infusion, decoction, dry plant tincture

- **Garlic**

THERAPEUTIC ACTION: Useful during epidemics; antibacterial, antiviral, enhances immunity; heals systemic and local infections, sore throats, staphylococcus and streptococcus infections

PREPARATION METHOD: Compress, immune compress for pneumonia and bronchitis; garlic compound (for upper respiratory infections or when fever is present, use garlic only as a compress)

- **Ginger**

  THERAPEUTIC ACTION: Antibacterial, antiviral, activates immunity

  PREPARATION METHOD: Standard hot infusion, fresh plant tincture, dry plant tincture, herbal wine

- **Green tea**

  THERAPEUTIC ACTION: Antiviral

  PREPARATION METHOD: Standard hot infusion

- **Lemon**

  THERAPEUTIC ACTION: Immune enhancer; useful during epidemics; clears toxins; antibacterial, antiviral, antihistamine, anti-inflammatory; heals pneumonia, bronchitis, fever

  PREPARATION METHOD: Fruit juice ($\frac{1}{2}$ lemon in 1 cup of water, drink 3 times per day)

- **Parsley**

  THERAPEUTIC ACTION: Antibacterial; antifungal; antihistamine; reduces fever

  PREPARATION METHOD: Standard hot infusion, decoction, fresh plant tincture, dry plant tincture, herbal compress

- **Sage**

  THERAPEUTIC ACTION: Immune enhancer; antifungal; antiviral

  PREPARATION METHOD: Standard hot infusion, standard cold infusion, decoction, fresh plant tincture, dry plant tincture, herbal bath

- **Savory**

  THERAPEUTIC ACTION: Immune enhancer; antibacterial; antifungal

  PREPARATION METHOD: Standard hot infusion, decoction, fresh plant tincture, dry plant tincture

- **Thyme**

  THERAPEUTIC ACTION: Strong antibiotic; reduces fever; soothes sore throat (as a gargle)

  PREPARATION METHOD: Standard hot infusion, decoction, fresh plant tincture, dry plant tincture

- **Turmeric**

  THERAPEUTIC ACTION: Anti-inflammatory; antibacterial; immune enhancer

  PREPARATION METHOD: Standard hot infusion, dry plant tincture

Foods

- **Cabbage**

  THERAPEUTIC ACTION: Antibacterial; anti-inflammatory

  PREPARATION METHOD: Vegetable compress, immune compress for pneumonia and bronchitis

Antiviral Foods

Apples, apple juice	Collards	Mushrooms
Barley	Cranberries	Orange juice
Black currants	Gooseberries	Peaches
Blueberries	Grapes	Pineapple juice
Chives	Lemon juice	Plums, plum juice

Antibacterial Foods

Apples	Chives	Mustard seed (black)
Bananas	Coconuts	Nutmeg
Beets	Cranberries	Olives
Blueberries	Cumin	Papayas
Cabbage	Dill	Plums
Carrots	Honey	Onions
Cashews	Horseradish	Sugar (cane sugar only)
Celery	Licorice	Watermelon
Chili peppers	Limes	Yogurt

Reflexology

For instructions on reflexology, see "Reflexology" under "How to Use the Therapy Section" at the beginning of Part II.

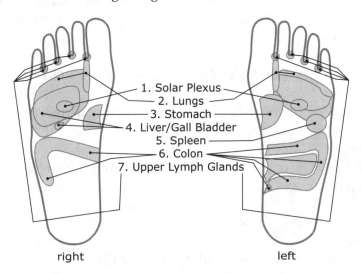

1. Solar Plexus
2. Lungs
3. Stomach
4. Liver/Gall Bladder
5. Spleen
6. Colon
7. Upper Lymph Glands

right   left

COUGHS AND RESPIRATORY AILMENTS

TEACHING

Coughs are caused by one of three factors: the cleansing of phlegm or toxins from the lung tissues; the movement of the respiratory diaphragm, which stimulates the gastric system, especially the stomach; or reactions to functional disturbances in the nerve system. In the following section, we will address these three factors from a Classical medicine perspective.

The Lungs and the Body's Systems

Classical medicine has always recognized a direct connection between the lungs and the intestines. In Chinese medicine, for example, the lungs and the large intestine are considered to be functional partners. The stomach also "controls" important aspects of the functions performed by the mucous membranes and the lungs. According to embryology, the lungs develop from the endoderm embryological tissue, which also produces the digestive organs. Therefore, we can think of the lungs as a "digestive" organ. The lungs' "digestion" is even evident in the first stages of digestive metabolism, when the energies and nutrients of the food we are metabolizing pass with the blood into the lungs and combine with the energies of the air we breathe, turning them into vital substances.

In the embryo, the lungs are formed from the endoderm tissues that create the large intestine. The large intestine and the lungs are very different organs, but have similar functions. By breathing in, the lungs take in the air that has been processed as a nutrient by the earth and its atmosphere and initiate the last stage of its metabolism. By breathing out, the lungs excrete the waste and toxins that are the byproducts of metabolism. Likewise, the large intestine initiates the last stage of digestion of food: it receives the nutrients from the digestive organs, further digests them, and excretes the final waste products from the body.

In the Classical medical traditions, a symptom like asthma is most often treated by stabilizing the functions of the stomach, which as mentioned above have a controlling effect on all mucous membranes as well as those of the lungs. Because the large intestine and the lungs are functional partners, chronic lung issues will affect the intestines, just as issues in the intestines will influence the functions of the lungs.

The upper respiratory tissues and sinuses along with the tissues of the mouth and throat are in reality extensions of our digestive system tissues. These oral cavity tissues are connected through the nose and lungs to the central nervous system in the brain. The Kidney/Bladder System also plays an important role in keeping the lung membranes clean and functioning. Thus, chronic kidney or bladder issues will compromise the lungs.

Lung tissues are compromised by airborne toxins, toxins located in the body and carried by the blood, and chronic problems in the digestive system, especially in the stomach and large intestine.

Air: The Universal Energy

Through the act of breathing, the lungs connect us to the entire cosmos and to the world around us. In Chinese medicine, the air we breathe is called "Ta Ch'i," meaning "the great universal energy." The air we breathe is the "breath" of the Earth and is composed of the energies found in the atmosphere as well as the energies of everything that grows and lives on the Earth. Air is one of the most life-giving of all nutrients. We can't live more than a very short time without breathing, whereas we can live a relatively long time without eating. We often think that only the oxygen in the air we breathe is important to our systems. Yet, if we breathed only pure oxygen we would die. The air we breathe is actually a complex nutrient containing subtle components of the Earth and atmosphere around us. These nutrients stimulate all mind-body processes. Living in areas with high levels of air pollution or in enclosed living spaces severely compromises our health. The modern so-called energy-efficient homes are built so tightly that minimal fresh air circulates in and out of them. Filtering used air merely cleans the particles from air. Fresh air, on the other hand, is constantly being revitalized by the earth and the atmosphere and becomes one of our most important nutrients.

Proper Breathing

Many health problems are associated with poor breathing patterns. When we breathe, it is important to do so mainly through the nose. The nose is directly connected energetically to the Large Intestine System, which means the process of digesting air begins in the nose. The nose has a series of mucous membranes that assist in this first stage of digestion. In addition to these membranes, the nose contains a special nerve system responsible for our sense of smell and for directly stimulating brain activity. These membranes also have immune cells that help healing processes in the sinuses. When we breathe through the nose, the in-rushing air stimulates these nerve centers and enhances our sense of smell, brain activities, and immune system functions.

The body's "breathing center," the energy system that controls the main aspects of respiration, is located in the middle of the breastbone, about even with the nipples of the breasts. At this point, virtually all of our bodily and mental functions unite. This breathing center is part of our rhythm system that ensures all bodily and mental processes remain stabile and in harmony with one another. Besides the lungs, the heart is the other major organ in this rhythm system. The regular beating of the heart and the rhythmical intake of our breath brings harmony to all the moments and events of our lives. We can see how the rhythm system is affected when we feel disturbed, frightened, or stressed. Our heartbeat changes and our breathing either becomes faster and more shallow or irregular. We can ease these feelings and gain a greater sense of harmony by taking a few deep breaths, which return our breathing and heartbeat to a normal rate. This rhythm system is also linked to our ability to move and use our limbs. The coordination involved in all our movements is reflected through the rhythmical functions of the lungs.

Another aspect of the lung-heart relationship appears in the circulation of the blood. The oxygen molecule that we breathe is the main carrier of the universal "Ta Ch'i" energies previously mentioned. Oxygen meets with the blood in the lung tissues and the energy from the "Ta Ch'i" (the air) vitalizes the blood. In the lungs, the oxygen also combines with the copper and iron found in our blood. Copper and iron are very important in nourishing the functions of all our cells and tissues and these minerals are one of the foundations of the immune system.

The sinuses are located around the front of the brain, eyes, and nose. The sinuses are open spaces or cavities in the bones of the skull. These cavities are connected to the breathing system and store the energies of the digested air very much like a battery. These energies fuel the brain, the senses, and their functions. In fact, all the cavities in our bodies that contain empty spaces store energy to help the body's tissues function correctly. The largest organ cavities in the body are the lungs and the large intestine. This fact underscores the important role that the Lung/Large Intestine System plays in building and maintaining the body's energy systems.

Emotions and the Lungs

Because the body and the mind are one integrated unit, emotions affect each organ. In the case of the lungs, grief is the main emotion that can compromise lung functions. Grief is a normal emotion yet, like all emotions, it needs healthy resources to resolve its impact. If grief is not resolved through appropriate spiritual and psychological resources and the patterns caused by grief continue into a chronic state, the lung functions will be compromised. Conversely, any set of factors that jeopardize lung functions can produce feelings of grief or inhibit the resolution of the grieving process.

THERAPY

Dry Coughs

Dry coughs usually involve chronic problems that fall outside the scope of this book. The following remedies, however, can still be used in the case of dry cough. Tissue salts, as well as reflexology, can be used as a supplemental treatment to whooping cough or for dry cough produced by other causes.

General Remedies

Remedy #1
- 8 ounces warm water
- 1 pinch of salt
- 2 pinches of turmeric powder (if available)

Gargle with 1 glass of warm water mixed with salt and turmeric powder (if you have it). This can be done several times a day.

Tissue Salts

Dryness of the throat
- *Natrum mur.* 6X

Dry coughs with sore and dry throat
- *Ferrum phos.* 6X

Dry, tickling cough with a feeling of constriction or tension in the throat
- *Mag. phos.* 6X

For all of the above, take the remedy 4–5 times per day for up to two days. Reduce the number of doses as symptoms improve.

Spices and Herbs

- **Basil**

  PREPARATION METHOD: Standard hot infusion, decoction, fresh plant tincture, dry plant tincture

- **Ginger**
  PREPARATION METHOD: Standard hot infusion, decoction, fresh plant tincture, dry plant tincture
- **Marjoram**
  PREPARATION METHOD: Standard hot infusion, decoction, fresh plant tincture, dry plant tincture
- **Thyme**
  PREPARATION METHOD: Standard hot infusion, decoction, fresh plant tincture, dry plant tincture

COUGH WITH PHLEGM (WITH OR WITHOUT FEVER)

These symptoms indicate that you might have bronchitis or pneumonia brought on by a cold or influenza. If the symptoms are *severe,* such as much rattling of mucus in the lungs and difficulty breathing, see your doctor or natural healthcare professional in addition to following these procedures.

The mucous membranes of the lungs and bronchia keep the tissues of our respiratory tract moist and active and play an important part in the chemistry of breathing. They also are related to the immune system, which keeps lung and bronchial tissues functioning well. When foreign substances like toxins or unwanted microbes come in contact with the mucous membranes, the immune system will create a cleansing and healing reaction. This produces heat and more mucus, which contains nutrients, immune substances, and dead or worn-out cells resulting from the healing processes. The immune system produces heat in the form of fever in local tissues as well as throughout the body. Fever initiates and speeds up healing and cleansing processes (see Coughs with Fever on page 95).

The bronchial tubes are lined with small hairlike structures that help move the extra mucus up to the throat and mouth so it can be coughed out and help the breathing. Nerve centers react to the presence of mucus and produce coughing.

The lungs and the large intestine work together as partners and support each other's functions. Healthy bowel function is very important for healthy lung function, and a condition like chronic constipation or irritable bowel syndrome will affect the lungs. According to Classical medicine, the natural time for bowel movements is between 5 A.M. and 7:30 A.M. In addition, the functions of both the kidneys and the stomach help to keep the lung membranes functioning correctly. Many chronic respiratory problems are due to disturbances in these organs. Respiration plays an important part in our digestive processes as well as building up our vitality, tissues, and immune system.

General Remedies

Remedy #1

- 1 cup finely chopped fresh, moist cabbage leaves
- 1 slice onion, finely chopped
- 1 clove of garlic, finely chopped

Make a compress for the lungs and bronchia, which will draw out toxins and strengthen the immune system. Combine cabbage, onion, and garlic. Chop further until all ingredients are very finely chopped, to a moist almost pastelike substance (or put in a blender or food processor).

Place the mixture on a single layer of cotton cloth or muslin, like a dish towel or other piece of material (without colors or patterns, which could contain irritants). Spread the mixture out in a large area at about the thickness of the little finger. Fold the cloth once to prevent the mixture from falling out, and place over the lungs and bronchia. Leave the compress on for 1 hour. Lift it off about every 15 minutes to see if the skin underneath is getting red. If this happens, remove the compress.

After 1 hour, or if the skin is getting red, remake the mixture using only cabbage and one small clove of garlic. This can be left on for 2 hours at a time. Replace with a fresh mixture of cabbage and garlic each time. A compress of only the cabbage can be left on all night.

For infants and small children, use $1/4$ onion slice and $1/4$ garlic clove. Check skin every five minutes when using the onion and garlic in the mixture.

Never use garlic internally when there is any fever or irritation of mucous membranes. Garlic is very good to use externally, however, under these same conditions.

Remedy #2

- 5 thin slices of fresh or $1/2$ teaspoon powdered ginger
- 1 cup of boiling water
- 1 pinch of powdered cloves (if available)
- 1 pinch of cinnamon
- $1/2$ teaspoon pure cane sugar

Make 1 cup of ginger tea. Fresh ginger should be cut into 5 thin slices about a half-inch in diameter, then chopped fine. Pour boiling water over the ginger and let it steep for 10 minutes. Drink when cool enough. If using powdered, mix ginger with boiling water. Drink 3 cups daily. This tea will help the immune system and all organ functions, especially the stomach, and will help eliminate mucus, which is important in respiratory problems. For a greater effect, add a pinch of cinnamon powder and/or powdered cloves to the ginger tea. If there is fever, you can add $\frac{1}{2}$ teaspoon of pure cane sugar. If only phlegm is present, add one teaspoon of honey (add honey only when tea is cool enough to drink). For children, cut down the amount of ginger.

Remedy #3
- 3 teaspoons each of chamomile, thyme, and/or dill
- 1 quart boiling water

Make an herbal bath by adding 1 quart (1 liter) of herbal tea made of chamomile, thyme, and dill. To make the tea, add any or all of these ingredients to the boiling water. Steep for 10 minutes. Pour into the bath water (at a temperature comfortable for you) and relax for 15 to 20 minutes.

Remedy #4
- Castor oil (fresh)

Rub castor oil on temples, palms, and soles of feet. This helps with phlegm.

Remedy #5
- 1 tablespoon honey
- 1 cup of warm water

Mix the honey in the warm water; drink 2–3 times daily to help expel phlegm.

Remedy #6
- 1 teaspoon of apple cider vinegar
- 1 glass of water

Mix apple cider vinegar in a glass of water. Drink in sips 2 times per day to help dissolve phlegm.

Remedy #7
- 1 glass of warm water
- 1 pinch of salt
- 2 pinches of turmeric powder (if available)

Gargle with the water mixed with the salt and the turmeric powder (if you have it). This can be done several times a day.

Tissue Salts
Clear Phlegm:
- *Ferrum phos* . 6X
- *Natrum mur.* 6X

Take these remedies together every hour up to 8 times; decrease the number of doses as symptoms begin to improve.

Whitish Phlegm:
- *Calc. phos.* 6X
- *Kali mur.* 6X

Take these remedies together every hour up to 8 times per day on the first day. Then, take every 2 hours up to 4 times for two to three days, if necessary; reduce the number of doses as symptoms begin to improve.

Greenish Phlegm:
- *Natrum sulph.* 6X
- *Kali sulph* 6X
- *Silicea* 6X

Take these remedies together every hour up to 8 times per day on the first day. Then, take every 2 hours up to 4 times for two to three days, if necessary; reduce the number of doses as symptoms begin to improve.

Yellowish Phlegm:
- *Calc. fluor.* 6X
- *Kali sulph.* 6X
- *Silicea* 6X
- *Calc. phos.* 6X
- *Kali phos.* 6X

Take these remedies together every hour up to 8 times per day on the first day. Then, take every 2 hours up to 4 times for 2–3 days, if necessary; reduce the number of doses as symptoms begin to improve.

Spices and Herbs

- **Anise seed**

  PREPARATION METHOD: Standard hot infusion, decoction, dry plant tincture
- **Basil**

  PREPARATION METHOD: Standard hot infusion, decoction, fresh plant tincture, dry plant tincture
- **Cayenne pepper**

  PREPARATION METHOD: Include in the diet. For sore throats in adults only, eat a mixture of a pinch of cayenne pepper with one teaspoon of honey.
- **Cinnamon**

  PREPARATION METHOD: Standard hot infusion, decoction, dry plant tincture
- **Fennel**

  PREPARATION METHOD: Standard hot infusion, decoction, dry plant tincture
- **Fenugreek**

  PREPARATION METHOD: Decoction, dry plant tincture

- **Garlic**
  PREPARATION METHOD: Garlic oil
- **Oregano**
  PREPARATION METHOD: Standard hot infusion, decoction, fresh plant tincture, dry plant tincture
- **Sage**
  PREPARATION METHOD: Standard hot infusion, decoction, fresh plant tincture, dry plant tincture
- **Thyme**
  PREPARATION METHOD: Standard hot infusion, decoction, fresh plant tincture, dry plant tincture

Foods

- **Carrots**
  PREPARATION METHOD: Include in the daily diet
- **Onions/leeks**
  PREPARATION METHOD I: Chop $\frac{1}{2}$ onion and simmer in 1 cup of water for 10 minutes. Cool to eating temperature and strain, reserving liquid. Add one tablespoon of honey to the liquid. Drink 1 cup 2–3 times daily.

  PREPARATION METHOD II: Chop onions into small pieces, cover in 1 inch of water, and simmer for 10 minutes. Add juice of $\frac{1}{2}$ lemon and simmer another 2–3 minutes. When cooled to eating temperature, strain and reserve the liquid. Add 1 teaspoon of honey to liquid and drink 1–3 times daily.

COUGHS WITH FEVER

Fever is not a disease—it is a natural response from the immune system and, like inflammation, it supports the body in its healing process. Fever brings heat, nutrients, and immune cells to all tissues, helping them to destroy unwanted microbes and cleanse the body of toxins. By increasing tissue metabolism, all of the body's processes function more quickly. Fever shows us that the immune system is working correctly and that the body needs to pause from its normal activities to concentrate on healing.

Children often develop higher fevers than adults. This is normal and does not mean that they are more ill. In the first ten years of life, the immune system is very active and cell metabolism is at its highest, allowing the body to build new tissues rapidly and to grow. High fevers usually break within twenty-four hours. When the fever breaks, the body usually sweats as it throws off toxins and cools itself. Give the child a lukewarm sponge bath over the entire body to cleanse and refresh the skin. Do not be alarmed by fever. It is a signal from the body that healing is taking place. If a fever is running extremely high (103°F) without falling for more than thirty-six hours and you have followed the procedures recommended, contact your physician.

You can help the fever to resolve itself (see "Fever" on page 164).

ASTHMATIC BREATHING OR DIFFICULTY IN BREATHING WITH NO FEVER/PHLEGM

Allergic reactions can impair breathing. Allergies are chronic (long-term) functional problems in the immune system. You can have an immune reaction to foods (so-called food allergies); to chemical toxins in your home, school, or work environment; to natural substances like pollen from plants and trees, and animal hair, among other things. Those things that you react to are not the *cause* of allergies. When the immune system reacts to a natural substance and causes a symptom to appear, it indicates that the immune system is out of balance and reacting in an inappropriate way. Allergies are usually the result of toxic effects on the body from such things as vaccinations, use of chemical medicines, or mercury fillings in the teeth.

Breathing is not only controlled by the function of the lungs, but also by a nerve center located in the brain stem. Often, the symptoms of asthma and allergic reactions reflect poor brain stem function. Asthma is not really a lung disease—it is only a symptom from other causes appearing in the lungs. The causes of asthma may be allergy patterns and toxins as mentioned above, chronic gastric disturbances (especially in the stomach), or problems occurring in the upper back or neck that affect the brain stem and the nerves that control the bronchia and respiration. See your natural healthcare professional for evaluation.

General Remedies

Remedy #1
- 5 thin slices fresh or $\frac{1}{2}$ teaspoon powdered ginger
- 1 cup of boiling water

Make a cup of ginger tea using either powdered or fresh ginger. Fresh ginger should be peeled and cut into five thin slices about a $\frac{1}{2}$-inch in diameter, then chopped fine. Pour boiling water over the ginger and let steep for 10 minutes. Drink when cool enough. If using powdered ginger, pour 1 cup of boiling water over $\frac{1}{2}$ teaspoon of ginger powder and let steep for 10 minutes. For children under age ten, use $\frac{1}{8}$ teaspoon ginger powder. If you have licorice powder, add one teaspoon to the infusion.

Drink 3 cups of ginger tea daily. This will help the immune system, all organ functions (especially the stomach), and help eliminate mucus, which is important to do in respiratory problems. For greater effect, add $\frac{1}{2}$ teaspoon of licorice powder and a pinch of cinnamon powder, and/or powdered cloves to the ginger tea. When fever is present, add $\frac{1}{2}$ teaspoon of pure cane sugar to the tea. If only phlegm is present, add 1 teaspoon of honey, being sure to add it when the tea is cool enough to drink.

Remedy #2
- $\frac{1}{2}$ teaspoon onion juice
- 1 teaspoon honey
- $\frac{1}{8}$ teaspoon black pepper

Mix onion juice with honey and the black pepper. Drink once daily for up to ten days. For children over age seven, dilute with water. *Do not give to children under seven years old.*

Tissue Salts
- *Kali phos.* 6X
- *Kali mur.* 6X
- *Mag. phos.* 6X
- *Natrum sulph.* 6X
- *Silicea* 6X

For acute symptoms, take these remedies together every hour up to 8 times for one to two days. Reduce the number of doses as symptoms begin to improve. For chronic symptoms, take remedies together 3 times daily for up to three weeks.

Spices, Herbs, and Foods
- **Anise seed**
  PREPARATION METHOD: Standard hot infusion, decoction, dry plant tincture
- **Basil**
  PREPARATION METHOD: Standard hot infusion, decoction, fresh plant tincture, dry plant tincture
- **Celery**
  PREPARATION METHOD: Include in the diet
- **Fennel**
  PREPARATION METHOD: Standard hot infusion, decoction, dry plant tincture
- **Garlic**
  PREPARATION METHOD: Garlic oil (apply externally to lung and bronchial area)

- **Ginger**

  PREPARATION METHOD: Standard hot infusion, decoction, fresh plant tincture, dry plant tincture

- **Marjoram**

  PREPARATION METHOD: Standard hot infusion, decoction, fresh plant tincture, dry plant tincture

- **Parsley**

  PREPARATION METHOD: Standard hot infusion, decoction, fresh plant tincture, dry plant tincture

- **Turmeric**

  PREPARATION METHOD: Decoction, dry plant tincture

UNCONTROLLABLE DRY COUGH FOLLOWED BY NOISY BREATH INTAKE AND/OR RUNNY NOSE AND SLIGHT TEMPERATURE

These symptoms indicate that your child may have whooping cough. See your doctor or natural healthcare professional if this is the case. The following therapies, however, will be a good supplement to any other therapies for whooping cough.

Tissue Salts

- *Mag. phos.* 6X

  Use this remedy in all cases, along with any of the remedies listed below when the symptoms they describe are present. Along with these tissue salts, follow the treatment for fever as well as the diet for coughs and respiratory ailments (listed below).

- *Calc. phos.* 6X—in cases where the child is teething

- *Ferrum phos.* 6X—during the first stage and/or when clear phlegm is present

- *Natrum mur.* 6X—in the first stages and/or when clear phlegm is present

- *Kali mur.* 6X—when there is a white coating on the tongue and/or when white phlegm is present

- *Kali sulph.* 6X—when yellowish phlegm is present

  For infants, dissolve 2 tablets of the appropriate tissue salt(s) in 1 teaspoon of water; mix and administer with a plastic (not metal) spoon. For children age three and older, give 4 tablets of the appropriate tissue salt(s) orally.

  On the first day, give 1 dose every ½ hour until any of the present symptoms change. Do not wake the child to give medicines. When *any* of the original symptoms *improve,* reduce the frequency of doses to 1 every 2 hours, but not for more than one day; then give dose 3 times daily for three additional days. When phlegm is present, change from one remedy to another if there are changes in the color of the phlegm (the phlegm color will indicate which remedy to use).

PRESSING PAIN IN FOREHEAD OR STUFFY NOSE WITH HEAVINESS IN THE FOREHEAD

This is a sign of a sinus headache. The main sinuses are located in the forehead and in the bones just below the eyes. Sinuses are empty spaces surrounded by bone and cartilage. They are lined with mucous membranes that are functional extensions of the membranes in the lungs and gastric areas. The sinuses are like reservoirs that hold and reflect the functional energies operating in the nose, eyes, and brain; they also act like a sounding chamber that gives tone and strength to our voice. The mucous membranes of the sinuses will tend to swell and produce mucus whenever factors affect the lungs or the intestines. The mucus will run down into the nose through small passages that connect the sinuses to the nose. If these are blocked from swelling, mucus will build up in the sinuses and cause pain. Sinus drainage can also cause a cough as the mucus runs down the back of the throat.

General Remedies

Remedy #1
- $\frac{1}{2}$ teaspoon sea salt (or regular salt)
- $\frac{1}{2}$ cup of lukewarm water

To make nose drops, dissolve sea salt (or regular salt) in water. Using an eyedropper, put six drops of the mixture in both nostrils, with the head held way back; keep the head tilted back for 30 seconds to allow the solution to run through the nasal cavities. You can do this 2–3 times a day.

Remedy #2
- $\frac{1}{2}$ teaspoon cinnamon
- $\frac{1}{2}$ teaspoon ginger
- 1 cup boiling water

Mix together the cinnamon, ginger, and boiling water. Let the mixture steep for 8 minutes. Dip a clean cloth into the mixture and use as a compress on the forehead; wring out the cloth and wet it again with more of the fresh mixture. Repeat every 5 minutes.

Tissue Salts

- *Kali mur.* 6X
- *Kali sulph.* 6X
- *Silicea* 6X

Take these remedies altogether 4 times daily; reduce the number of dosages as symptoms improve.

Spices, Herbs, and Foods

- **Black pepper**
  PREPARATION METHOD: Dry plant tincture; include in the daily diet
- **Cardamom**
  PREPARATION METHOD: Standard hot infusion, decoction, dry plant tincture
- **Cinnamon**
  PREPARATION METHOD: Standard hot infusion, decoction, dry plant tincture
- **Fennel**
  PREPARATION METHOD: Standard hot infusion, decoction, dry plant tincture
- **Ginger**
  PREPARATION METHOD: Standard hot infusion, decoction, fresh plant tincture, dry plant tincture
- **Sage**
  PREPARATION METHOD: Standard hot infusion, decoction, fresh plant tincture, dry plant tincture

GENERAL DIET FOR COUGHS AND RESPIRATORY AILMENTS

Recommended Foods

- Apple (grated or juice)
- Avocado
- Broccoli (lightly cooked)
- Cabbage (lightly boiled)
- Carrot juice or grated carrot with every meal, if possible
- Cranberry (medium cooked or juice)
- Green pepper (cooked/baked/stir-fried)
- Honey
- Kale (steamed/medium boiled/stir-fried)
- Olive oil (in stir-frying)
- Onions (boiled/stir-fried/baked)
- Orange juice
- Parsley raw or lightly boiled with every meal, if possible

- Pineapple juice
- Potato (mashed)
- Red grapes (juice)
- Rice (boiled well)
- Spinach (lightly cooked/stir-fried)
- Unprocessed cane sugar (only a little)

Foods to Avoid

- Additives, preservatives, MSG, colorings, and artificial flavors
- Caffeine
- Corn oil, safflower oil, sunflower oil
- Dairy products
- Eggs
- Meats
- Oats
- Peanuts
- Processed sugars
- Soy products
- Wheat products

Spices and Herbs

- **Anise seed**

  THERAPEUTIC ACTION: Expels phlegm; opens chest; relieves wheezing and asthmatic breathing

  PREPARATION METHOD: Standard hot infusion, decoction, dry plant tincture

- **Basil**

  THERAPEUTIC ACTION: Expels phlegm; relieves wheezing, spasmodic cough, asthma, whooping cough, and sinusitis

  PREPARATION METHOD: Standard hot infusion, decoction, fresh plant tincture, dry plant tincture

- **Black pepper**

  THERAPEUTIC ACTION: Relieves coughing and nasal irritation

  PREPARATION METHOD: Dry plant tincture; include in the daily diet

- **Cardamom**

  THERAPEUTIC ACTION: Expels phlegm; relieves sinusitis and chronic bronchitis

  PREPARATION METHOD: Standard hot infusion, decoction, dry plant tincture

- **Cayenne pepper**

  THERAPEUTIC ACTION: Relieves sore throats, hoarseness, laryngitis, and acute and chronic bronchitis

PREPARATION METHOD: Include in the diet; for sore throats (in adults only), eat a mixture of a pinch of cayenne pepper with one teaspoon of honey

- **Cinnamon**

  THERAPEUTIC ACTION: Relieves bronchitis and upper respiratory problems

  PREPARATION METHOD: Standard hot infusion, decoction, dry plant tincture

- **Fennel seed**

  THERAPEUTIC ACTION: Stimulates lungs; expels phlegm; opens chest; relieves wheezing, asthma, and hoarseness

  PREPARATION METHOD: Standard hot infusion, decoction, dry plant tincture

- **Fenugreek seed**

  THERAPEUTIC ACTION: Expels phlegm; antibiotic

  PREPARATION METHOD: Decoction, dry plant tincture

- **Garlic**

  THERAPEUTIC ACTION: Antiviral and antibacterial; expels phlegm; opens chest; relieves wheezing, bronchitis, and asthma

  PREPARATION METHOD: Garlic oil (apply externally to lung and bronchial area)

- **Ginger**

  THERAPEUTIC ACTION: Expels phlegm; relieves asthma; anti-inflammatory; relieves whooping cough

  PREPARATION METHOD: Standard hot infusion, decoction, fresh plant tincture, dry plant tincture

- **Marjoram**

  THERAPEUTIC ACTION: Relieves asthma and violent coughing

  PREPARATION METHOD: Standard hot infusion, decoction, fresh plant tincture, dry plant tincture

- **Oregano**

  THERAPEUTIC ACTION: Immune enhancer; good for bronchitis

  PREPARATION METHOD: Standard hot infusion, decoction, fresh plant tincture, dry plant tincture

- **Parsley**

  THERAPEUTIC ACTION: Relieves coughs and asthma

  PREPARATION METHOD: Standard hot infusion, decoction, fresh plant tincture, dry plant tincture

- **Rosemary**

  THERAPEUTIC ACTION: Relieves asthma

  PREPARATION METHOD: Standard hot infusion, decoction, fresh plant tincture, dry plant tincture

- **Sage**
  THERAPEUTIC ACTION: Stimulates lung functions; expels phlegm; acts as anti-microbial
  PREPARATION METHOD: Standard hot infusion, decoction, fresh plant tincture, dry plant tincture
- **Thyme**
  THERAPEUTIC ACTION: Expels phlegm; antibiotic; relieves laryngitis; helps whooping cough and spasmodic coughing
  PREPARATION METHOD: Standard hot infusion, decoction, fresh plant tincture, dry plant tincture
- **Turmeric**
  THERAPEUTIC ACTION: Relieves asthma
  PREPARATION METHOD: Decoction, dry plant tincture

Foods

- **Carrots**
  THERAPEUTIC ACTION: Relieves chronic bronchitis
  PREPARATION METHOD: Include in the daily diet
- **Celery**
  THERAPEUTIC ACTION: Relieves asthma, wheezing, and hoarseness
  PREPARATION METHOD: Include in the diet
- **Chicory**
  THERAPEUTIC ACTION: Expels phlegm
  PREPARATION METHOD: Standard hot infusion, decoction, fresh plant tincture, dry plant tincture
- **Honey and lemon**
  THERAPEUTIC ACTION: Relieves coughs and sore throats
  PREPARATION METHOD: Drink 1 cup warm, unsweetened lemonade made from fresh lemons with 1 teaspoon of honey added. To make a cough syrup, mix 1 part honey with 1 part lemon juice; take 1 teaspoon every 2–3 hours.
- **Onions/leeks**
  THERAPEUTIC ACTION: Relieves coughs and asthma; reduces phlegm
  PREPARATION METHOD I: Chop $1/2$ onion and simmer in 1 cup of water for 10 minutes. Cool to eating temperature and strain, reserving liquid. Add 1 tablespoon of honey to the liquid. Drink 1 cup 2–3 times daily.
  PREPARATION METHOD II: Chop onions into small pieces, cover in 1 inch of water, and simmer for 10 minutes. Add juice of $1/2$ lemon and simmer another 2–3 minutes. When cooled to eating temperature, strain and reserve the liquid. Add 1 teaspoon of honey to liquid. Drink 1–3 times daily.

Immune Poultice for Pneumonia and Bronchitis:

- 2 cups white cabbage
- 1 slice from center of medium-large onion
- 1 slice from a clove of garlic
- 1 piece of white, bandanna-size cotton

Finely chop white cabbage to an almost mushlike state. The finished amount should equal a small handful. Chop onion to the same consistency as the cabbage. Do the same with the garlic. Mix the ingredients. Spread the juicy mixture on $\frac{1}{2}$ of the cotton (bandanna size); fold the other half over mixture to keep it in place. Lay the poultice on the lung/bronchial area and leave in place for 1 hour, but check every 15 minutes. If redness develops or there is heat under the poultice, remove it. After removal, wash the area with clean water. Then, remake the poultice, without the onion. Leave the poultice on for the rest of the hour.

Decongestants:

Use the following in the diet: chili, garlic, horseradish, mustard, onion, black pepper, thyme, and chamomile tea with grated ginger

Reflexology

For instructions on reflexology, see "Reflexology" under "How to Use the Therapy Section" at the beginning of Part II.

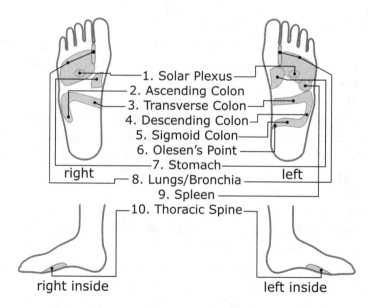

1. Solar Plexus
2. Ascending Colon
3. Transverse Colon
4. Descending Colon
5. Sigmoid Colon
6. Olesen's Point
7. Stomach
8. Lungs/Bronchia
9. Spleen
10. Thoracic Spine

right   left

right inside   left inside

DENTAL HEALTH

TEACHING

Our teeth represent one of the most neglected and misunderstood systems of the body. This is unfortunate because the oral cavity (mouth) plays an extremely important role in the health of our bodies and all of its functions. Although current dental practice is becoming more and more technically advanced, it sorely lacks an understanding of the influence that the teeth and gums exert on the health of the whole body.

Although the concept of dental care with frequent checkups has been in place for the last fifty years, the dental profession still treats the teeth as more or less external parts of the body, used only for chewing food and enhancing our smile. As such, teeth can be repaired as you might repair a mechanical appliance. Not understanding the role that the teeth play in our health and the deeper functions of our organ systems has contributed to serious chronic health problems. Many health issues like heart disease and arthritis can be caused by problems originally related to the teeth.

The Teeth and the Embryological Tissues

The teeth are developed from two of the three embryological tissue systems, which gives us the first clue as to the role teeth play in our body. The outer tissue of the tooth, called the enamel, develops from the ectoderm embryological tissue. This tissue also creates the brain and nerve system. The ectoderm is the "energy network" behind the functioning of all of our senses, and it also creates the nerve pathways to all tissues and organs. Tooth enamel begins to develop when the embryo is only six weeks old. Such early development indicates that the teeth are connected to, and play a role in, the nerve tissue and sensory functions of the developing fetal child. This role continues throughout life. Anything compromising the tooth enamel will interfere with the Nerve/Sense System and its functions.

The tooth's pulp, along with its other anatomical features, is developed from the mesoderm embryological tissue system. The mesoderm creates the heart, kidneys, connective tissue, bones, muscles, blood, and lymph. The mesoderm organs and tissues control and integrate the "rhythms" of all the body and mind functions. The tissues and organs of this system stabilize and harmonize these functions so that they work well together. Since the tooth pulp is part of the mesoderm system, it contributes to the harmony and stability of the body's functions. Anything compromising the tooth pulp will interfere with the mesoderm tissue system and its functions.

The roots of the teeth are controlled by the energies of the Stomach System. This connection underscores the great wisdom of nature. When we chew, we automatically stimulate the first primary organ in our digestive system, the stomach, which in turn initiates our entire digestive process. This happens because the joint of the jaw, the temporomandibular joint (TMJ), is controlled by the energies of the Stomach System. These energies are activated by chewing, which stimulates the stomach's functions.

The oral cavity containing the teeth and gums is connected energetically to the functions of all the pelvic organs, including the reproductive organs, the kidney and bladder, and the colon. The oral cavity and the pelvic organs mirror one another, meaning that the problems of the one will affect the other. Likewise, resolving problems in the one will support the other.

The mucous membranes of the oral cavity are an extension of the digestive tract membranes. We must remember that our digestive system is like one long tube, starting in the mouth, extending through the body, and ending at the anus. The oral cavity, therefore, is an important part of our digestive system and the health of the oral cavity directly affects our body's ability to nourish itself.

The Problems with Root Canals

When the living part of the tooth, the pulp, is severely damaged or invaded by decay, the tooth will die and infection may spread to the jawbone tissue. A root canal is a dental procedure used to resolve the infection and prevent having to extract the tooth. At first glance, this procedure seems logical, but the chronic health problems created by root canals far outweigh their advantages.

The root canal procedure removes all of the nerves and blood/lymph vessels that extend from the tooth's root to the pulp. In a healthy state, these nerves and vessels provide nourishment to the pulp. The empty root is then filled with a material to prevent the empty cavity from forming bacteria that will inflame the surrounding ligament and bone. Removing the nerve and vascular tissues kills the tooth and stops the inflammation caused by the decay, and also alleviates the pain caused by the inflamed nerves. This procedure allows the tooth to remain in place, though it is no longer living or biologically integrated in the body's systems. One of the problems with root canals is that the body will always try to reject and "clean out" the presence of dead tissues in its ligaments and bones. It's like having a splinter in your finger that you can't remove—the body will eventually reject the splinter on its own.

A more serious problem is that the materials used to fill the root canal have particles that are too big to fill the small tubules, or channels, extending from the main canal into the tooth pulp. Thus, they remain open and bacteria develop in them. One of the main bacteria that forms in these spaces is the same bacteria involved with Lyme disease. The bacteria in a root canal mutate, however, and shed their cell walls and therefore do not stimulate the immune system to initiate a healing process. These pathological bacteria then move throughout the body's systems creating the basis for many chronic diseases, including heart disease and arthritis. These and other chronic diseases are considered to be isolated problems by the medical profession. Conventional doctors never look at the possibility of these pathologies being connected to the teeth. Natural medical practitioners often find that when they recommend the extraction of a tooth that has a root canal, other health issues are resolved.

The concept behind root canals directly opposes nature's way of dealing with seriously diseased teeth. If we look at the anatomy of the jawbone, we see that the teeth are not directly part of the bone. Rather, they are suspended like hammocks in the bone pocket by small ligaments that hold the teeth in place. In the wisdom of nature, increasing inflammation and infection causes a tooth to loosen so that it can fall out. A dentist can facilitate this by pulling the tooth. Contradicting nature's law by keeping a dead tooth in the mouth at any cost is a bad idea. A badly infected tooth (or a nonliving root canal tooth) is a health hazard to the body due to the fact that the toxins from infection go directly into the bloodstream and are carried throughout the body causing secondary problems. In addition, research has shown that each tooth has an energetic connection to a specific set of organs and tissues. A diseased tooth will directly affect and compromise those particular systems to which it is connected through its energy reflexes.

Cavities and Amalgam Fillings

Cavities are spots of degeneration in the tooth enamel and are created in two ways. First, through improper nutrition or problems with the digestive process, the tooth pulp is not properly nourished, causing degenerative processes in the enamel and other parts of the tooth. It is a myth, however, that sugar by itself causes tooth decay. Most sweets like candy, ice cream, and commercial snacks are made from processed sugars and contain additives that create problems in digestive processes and impair the function of tissues including teeth enamel. Processed sweets increase tissue metabolism; this increased metabolism can ultimately degenerate tissues because the tissues are forced to use their own substances as nutrients. People who eat a lot of sweets usually have poor diets. A craving for sweets always indicates chronic problems in the primary digestive metabolism as a whole as well as physical or emotional stress; these problems will always affect the teeth.

Second, cavities result from stressors in the nerve system. Remember, the tooth enamel is created from the same embryological tissue, the ectoderm, as the brain and the nerves. Chronic stress contributes to the degeneration of tissues including tooth enamel, which eventually can result in cavities. To deal with the *cause* of cavities, it is vital to make sure that the digestive processes and nutrition are in order and that chronic stress in the nerve system has been resolved.

When dentists find a cavity, they usually fill it. This is a relatively simple procedure and is not very invasive. The spot of decay on the enamel is drilled out and cleaned down to the healthy tissue, and the hole is filled with a material to strengthen the tooth. However, two problems can occur with filling the teeth. One minor concern is that in the event of a deep cavity, if the drilling is not done properly, the procedure may damage the pulp, causing the tooth to die. The main problem, however, pertains to the choice of filling material.

For almost a century, dentists have used amalgam fillings, a mixture of metals that includes mercury as a main ingredient. Considerable research has shown mercury to be highly toxic. It damages the functions of the liver and kidneys, affects the entire intestinal tract, and compromises the digestive process as well as the metabolic energies of the kidney. Moreover, it strongly inhibits the immune system's functions and the body's healing processes.

Mercury is a heavy metal that always seeks the tissues that have the highest metabolism, such as the liver, kidneys, and intestinal tract. If a pregnant woman has mercury fillings, the mercury toxins will be drawn directly to the fetus because the fetus has a higher metabolic rate than any other of the mother's own tissues. This means that the infant is born with mercury toxicity, which it will have to cleanse from its system in order to develop healthfully. Natural health practitioners often find that when dealing with young children's health problems, and those of adults as well, they need to cleanse the mercury out of their systems before they can fully resolve the particular health issue.

Mercury toxins cannot be removed permanently from the body as long as the mercury fillings remain. Ultimately, the amalgams should be replaced by a biologically compatible material. Over the last forty years, the dental industry has developed a number of options for filling material, all of which are better than mercury. Yet, a number of them are made from compounds that affect the hormone system or are slowly dissolved by the natural digestive substances found in the mouth. Consult a competent natural healthcare professional about which options are best for you.

The Dangers of Fluoride

Dentists have long promoted the use of fluoride to prevent tooth decay. The fluoride used in this way differs from the fluoride that the body produces, and it is highly toxic. Although fluoride makes tooth enamel strong and durable, the body's natural fluoride is a *calcium fluoride,* not the inorganic product used in the dental industry. This commercial fluoride affects the natural growth process in bones and cartilage, and compromises the digestive system as well. The fluoride used by dentists is toxic to the system (which is why they say not to swallow it). This is also true of fluoridated water, which is used in most American communities, and of fluoride in toothpastes. Calcium fluoride found naturally in the body is essential for creating strong tissues and bones. The fluoride used in the dental and medical industries significantly contributes to poor health because it interferes with the digestive metabolism of protein needed for building strong tissues. In addition, fluoride weakens the immune system, making us vulnerable to serious disease and interfering with our ability to integrate our physiological and mental activities.

THERAPY

BLEEDING GUMS

General Remedies

Remedy #1
- Juice of $\frac{1}{2}$ lemon
- 1 cup water
- 1 pinch of salt
  Mix the lemon juice into 1 cup of water. Add a pinch of salt and drink.

Remedy #2
- $\frac{1}{2}$ teaspoon salt
- 1 cup warm water
  Dissolve salt in a glass of warm water. Swish around in the mouth twice daily.

Tissue Salts
- *Calc. sulph.* 6X

- *Calc. phos.* 6X
- *Natrum mur.* 6X
- *Kali phos.* 6X

Take these remedies together 3 times daily for up to three weeks. Pause for three weeks, then repeat the cycle, if necessary.

TOOTHACHE

Herbal Remedy

- 3 drops of clove oil

Place clove oil on a cotton ball. Apply to gum of the tooth. Leave in place $\frac{1}{2}$ hour. Repeat 3–4 times per day.

Tissue Salts

- *Silicea* 6X
- *Mag. phos.* 6X
- *Calc. phos.* 6X
- *Kali mur.* 6X
- *Calc. fluor.* 6X
- *Kali phos.* 6X

Take these remedies together 3–5 times daily for acute toothache. Reduce the number of doses as symptoms begin to improve. For a chronic tendency to toothache, take the remedies together 3 times daily for up to three weeks.

Spices, Herbs, and Foods

- **Caraway**
  PREPARATION METHOD: Herbal compress, herbal oil
- **Clove**
  PREPARATION METHOD: Herbal oil (Prepare oil by filling a small jar with bruised cloves. Cover with olive oil. After one week, strain out cloves and save the oil in the refrigerator; repeat process by adding a new batch of bruised cloves to the oil. The oil will stay fresh for two weeks.)
- **Garlic**
  PREPARATION METHOD: Herbal oil, garlic oil
- **Ginger**
  PREPARATION METHOD: Herbal oil (Prepare oil by filling a small jar with pieces of fresh ginger. Cover with olive oil; after one week, strain out the ginger and save the oil.)
- **Thyme**
  PREPARATION METHODS: Herbal oil, herbal compress

- **Turmeric**

  PREPARATION METHOD: Take 1 teaspoon of turmeric twice daily with food.

RECEDING GUMS

Tissue Salts

- *Calc. phos.* 6X
- *Kali phos.* 6X
- *Kali mur.* 6X

  Take these remedies together twice per day for up to three weeks.

TO NOURISH TEETH AND PREVENT DECAY

Tissue Salts

- *Calc. phos.* 6X
- *Calc. fluor.* 6X
- *Silicea* 6X

  Take these remedies together twice per day for 4 weeks.

GENERAL CARE OF THE TEETH

Spices, Herbs, and Foods

- **Caraway**

  THERAPEUTIC ACTION: Antibiotic; relieves toothache

  PREPARATION METHOD: Herbal compress, herbal oil

- **Clove**

  THERAPEUTIC ACTION: Antiplaque; anesthetic for toothache

  PREPARATION METHOD: Herbal oil (Prepare oil by filling a small jar with bruised cloves. Cover with olive oil. After one week, strain out cloves and save the oil in the refrigerator; repeat process by adding a new batch of bruised cloves to the oil. The oil will stay fresh for two weeks.)

- **Garlic**

  THERAPEUTIC ACTION: Antibiotic; relieves toothache

  PREPARATION METHOD: Garlic oil

- **Ginger**

  THERAPEUTIC ACTION: Alleviates toothache

  PREPARATION METHOD: Herbal oil (Prepare oil by filling a small jar with pieces of fresh ginger. Cover with olive oil; after one week, strain out the ginger and save the oil.)

- **Thyme**
  THERAPEUTIC ACTION: Antibiotic; relieves toothache
  PREPARATION METHOD: Herbal oil, herbal compress
- **Turmeric**
  THERAPEUTIC ACTION: Antibiotic; restores tissues; relieves toothache
  PREPARATION METHOD: Take $\frac{1}{4}$ teaspoon of turmeric twice daily with food

  Natural Toothpaste: Mix equal amounts of salt and baking soda.
  Wet your toothbrush, dip into the mixture, and brush well.

Reflexology

For instructions on reflexology, see "Reflexology" under "How to Use the Therapy Section" at the beginning of Part II.

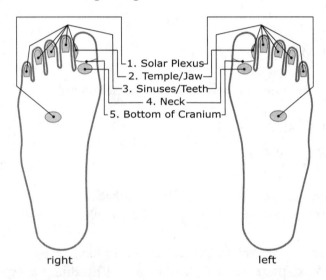

1. Solar Plexus
2. Temple/Jaw
3. Sinuses/Teeth
4. Neck
5. Bottom of Cranium

right   left

DIGESTIVE DYSFUNCTION

TEACHING

The digestive system is an infinitely complex alchemist's laboratory of living tissues and energies as powerful as the sun. At every moment, our digestive system is transforming the life of the universe into the form of our cells, the life of our tissues, and the sweep of our emotions. As we have mentioned, this process is termed *metabolism,* from the original Greek word meaning "transformation of matter."

Metabolism: Change and Transformation

For a moment, let's broaden the typical conception we have of metabolism. We all know that our bodies metabolize the food we eat, the air that we breathe, and the water we drink, along with everything else that we take in to nourish us and keep us alive. Food, air, and water are composed of the same matter and energy as the stars in distant galaxies, the sun and the planets of our solar system, and the soil of the Earth. When we eat, drink, or breathe, we are being nourished by the matter and energy that continually create and maintain the entire universe. We can see this nourishment happening all around us as we observe nature recreating itself through constant change and transformation. In fact, we could say that the only constant in reality is change and its transformations.

This process of change and transformation is what the word *metabolism* means. Digestion is the most fundamental expression of the metabolic process. Our own digestive process is but a single stage of a universal metabolic process of transformation and creation taking place throughout the entire universe. The carrot we eat, for example, did not suddenly appear out of nothing but is a manifestation of these transformative metabolic processes working throughout the universe.

At first glance, this concept is very difficult to grasp, mostly due to our inexperience of using simple observable facts to understand that which *appears* to be hopelessly complex. Let's return to the example of the carrot. If we use a short version of how the carrot came to be, we could say that the sun metabolizes its own matter into light and heat. Heat and light profoundly affect the Earth's fertile soil and the atmosphere's moisture. Light and heat transform soil and moisture into nutrients. The creative metabolic powers inherent in a carrot seed use and transform the matter and energy found in the soil, which has been fertilized by the atmosphere and the sun, to grow into a carrot. Because nature is a continual process of transformation and change, at some point this carrot will undergo a radical metabolic transformation. Either it will be eaten and completely transformed by the digestive process of an animal or human, or it will wither and die in the field and be digested and transformed by the energies of the soil itself.

The important point to understand about metabolism is that everything we take into the body from the outside is foreign to us. A carrot, a piece of meat, or an apple all have their own individual biological systems and are specific forms of life that differ from ours. The daily miracle involved in digestion is that our body consumes this foreign matter and *transforms* it into the cells and processes of the body, a body with its own unique identity and purpose.

Our food is made up of the atomic fires of the stars; the crystal patterns that give form to the planets, shells, rock, and bones; the complex biochemistry that takes place in the roots, leaves, and flowers of plants; and the stabilizing chemistry found in the flesh of the meat we eat. We are all part of a transforming metabolic process that both nourishes us and fulfills the destiny of our lives.

We often forget that metabolism—the transforming of matter into our own life—happens not just with food, but also with impressions and experiences, which means that our minds and their thoughts also are part of the digestive process. In order for our minds to think and feel, we must digest impressions and thoughts. When thinking over a situation, we sometimes say, "Let me digest that." We think and feel with our digestion as much as we do with our brains. In fact, the nerves of our brains do not think, they merely relay signals back and forth between body systems as we "digest" our impressions and experiences into new thoughts and feelings, just as we transform food into our own cells and tissues. In reality, we think and feel through the functions of the organ systems that control our metabolic and digestive processes. The brain is somewhat like a computer—it receives commands and inputs information from all of the body's systems and processes; it then works as a relay network that passes this information to tissues and organs and causes them to respond to the message.

Digestion as Renewal

Our digestive processes also renew us. In our tissues, thousands of cells die every second and new cells are created to replace them. Our digestive metabolism accomplishes this rejuvenation. The same process occurs in our minds. One thought dies and is replaced by a new one. We call this digestive process "thinking." Thinking is a creative process, and creative processes always form new things, both new thoughts and new cells.

Even our vision is a process of digestion. We have the ability to see because objects around us reflect light onto a part of the eye called the retina, which is covered by a special tissue that is chemically sensitive to light. This light-sensitive tissue digests the light, turning it into biochemical components that stimulate nerve tissues in the back of the retina and move through these nerve endings to brain areas that produce image impressions. This biochemical process is related to the same process that occurs in the stomach and intestines when digesting food; in fact, the liver, which plays an important role in our digestion, also controls the light-sensitive biochemical processes and nerve response in the retina of the eye.

We are constantly changing, maturing, and growing in body and mind. We are not completely the same now as we were five minutes ago. We are being renewed and reformed every second by life. The ability to live and grow is a deep and complex process of metabolism. People often say "you are what you eat," although in reality we can say you are what you digest, what you metabolize.

The Embryological Systems and Digestion

The cells and tissues that govern metabolism, the foundation of digestion and nutrition, are the first cells to form in the embryo in the mother's womb. In order for the embryo to grow and develop, it needs to transform the outer world of food, water, and air, into a body that can live, feel, think, and recreate itself. These cells, which begin to form in the first few days following conception, become the endoderm, one of the three original tissues of our embryonic body. The endoderm tissue develops into our digestive organs. This tissue system has the ability to transform matter into energy and develop the very foundation of who we are and who we become in our physical and mental being.

The endoderm embryological system controls the metabolic and digestive processes. The hormone glands produced by the endoderm make up the other major communication network of the digestive process. Hormones are messengers like the nerves of the body. Just as the nerve system has the brain as a central gathering and relay organ, so the hormone system has a similar central system in the pineal gland, hypothalamus gland, and liver, all of which receive information on hormonal activity from the body's systems. This system coordinates the gathered information and sends hormonal messages out to the other glands, tissues, and organs causing them to respond.

The Energies of Digestion

Digestive metabolism is governed by energies rather than by chemistry. All of the biochemicals that we can identify in our digestive process are produced by the energies inherent in our food, water, and the air we breathe. In the Classical medical traditions, these energies are referred to as "Tastes." We might think that this word refers to whether something tastes sweet or salty or bitter, but in a medical context, Taste refers to the energies in food. Everything in nature is composed of varying combinations of energetic properties called Elements—Earth, Water, Fire, Air, and Space. These Elements influence all our tissues and their processes. For example, the predominance of the Water and Fire Elements produces the Salty Taste; salt itself is made up primarily of these two energies. Conversely, a predominance of Water and Earth energies will produce the Sweet Taste, of which sugar is a good example. Our digestion unlocks these energies in foods. This unlocking of and utilization of energies defines the process of *nutrition.*

All foods consist of their own tissues and biochemical substances, organized in such a way as to make that particular food unique. Although all things embody the same primary Elements, the *specific* combinations of these Elements produce unique forms of life. Obviously a great difference in life forms exists between a carrot and a human being. For us to gain any nutrition from a life form so different and foreign to us, we need to be able not only to digest it but also to transform its life energies into our own unique human energy patterns.

When we eat and digest a carrot, the carrot is completely burned up by our metabolism in the organs responsible for digestion. We can understand this process if we watch a log being burned in a campfire. The log is completely transformed (digested) by fire into its primary energies of heat and light, leaving only ash. The energy of heat and light inherent in the life form of wood that make up the log's tissues is released, while the remaining ash is reabsorbed into the earth.

Our digestion works in a similar way. It breaks food down into its energy components. The released energy is then used by our body to create vital nutrients that in turn create new cells and tissues. The waste products, which are equivalent to the ash from the burned log, are eliminated from our bodies in the form of vapor emitted from our lungs and skin, as well as in the form of urine and feces.

If we could track a molecule of the mineral phosphorus found in the carrot we're eating, we would notice that at a particular point during the digestive process, the molecule would completely disappear. The fire of our metabolic processes would completely burn it up. The energy released from the metabolic process would be used by the body, in this case to construct a molecule of a substance needed to support its functions. If, for example, our body needed magnesium rather than phosphorus but we were only eating phosphorus, the digestive process would use the energy released from the metabolized phosphorus to create magnesium.

The Digestive Processes

Digestion actually begins with the sight, thought, and smell of food. When we are hungry and think of, see, or smell an appealing food, we begin to secrete more saliva. Saliva contains digestive enzymes that start the process of digestion and metabolism in our mouths with the first bite. The food already being digested then travels down to the stomach.

Our digestive system, often called the gastrointestinal (GI) tract in conventional medicine, is a long tube of tissues and organs—the largest single system in our body, stretching from the mouth to the anus. As previously mentioned, it is created by the embryological tissue called the endoderm, which also creates the glands and the inner surface of the lungs.

The stomach governs the digestion of all primary nutrients that build cells and tissues. These nutrients belong to the Sweet Taste energies like sugars, gluten, and carbohydrates. The Stomach System works together with the spleen and pancreas. These organs are also directly connected to the feeling of well-being in the psyche; to the functions of the lymph system and blood plasma; to the production of milk during pregnancy; to the immune system functions; and to menstruation in women. The Classical medical traditions think of an organ as being not just a specific organ in an anatomical sense but as being a complex system of functions that the organ controls.

From the stomach, the partially digested food moves into the small intestine, where it is further digested. The nutrient products resulting from this stage of digestion are absorbed into the wall of the small intestine through tiny fingerlike tissues called *villi* and are then transported by the blood to the liver.

The liver is one of the most complex of all metabolic organs. It produces the bile that is stored in the gallbladder and, from there, pumped into the first part of the small intestine called the duodenum, where the second stage of digestion begins. Bile helps metabolize fats, activates pancreatic digestive enzymes, and absorbs cholesterol.

Besides these activities, the liver plays a very important role in the immune system. Immune cells in the liver protect the body against microbes that the body has no immediate use for and help the body deal with destructive toxins. The liver also serves as the first stage in establishing balance in the hormone system. It measures the hormonal content of the blood and sends signals via the circulation to the gland called the hypothalamus, which functions as a master control system for the hormones. Classical medicine also recognizes that the liver's domain extends to the function of the eyes and the midbrain, as well as controlling certain functions of the muscles, tendons, and joints.

The large intestine is involved in the final stage of digestion. Membranes in the colon absorb the last fluid nutrients from the food that has passed through all earlier stages of digestion and allows them to circulate in the blood. The large intestine is also directly connected to the functions of the central nerve system in the brain and the autonomic nerve system that provides nerve signals for the body's organs. The movement of food through the large intestine stimulates a network of nerves that cover the outer intestinal walls, and this network of nerves in turn stimulates these other systems. The digestive process in the large intestine influences our emotional life as well. There is a nerve bundle in the intestinal muscle of the rectum of the large intestine that signals the brain when it is time to have a bowel movement. This same nerve bundle is very sensitive to emotional stress, which can impair its functions. This is why we often experience constipation when under emotional stress and why regular bowel movements help maintain stability in our emotional lives. The process of digestion and the transformation of food is an event controlled by the functional energies of several important organ systems as well as by the biochemical processes found in the intestinal tract. The GI tract provides the biochemical components of digestion. The Kidney System and the reproductive organs provide the subtle functional energies for making the biochemical transformations possible. This is why caring for the kidneys supports the digestive processes. When these functions are impaired, incomplete digestion will occur, resulting in malnourished cells and tissues, as well as increased biotoxins. These biotoxins are absorbed by the mucous membranes of the intestines and enter the bloodstream, compromising the body's tissues.

The Lung System also plays an important role in digestion by directing the energies of the oxygen we breathe into the metabolic process. This oxidizing process can be observed in nature when we see a piece of iron rusting. The oxygen of the air works as a digesting agent, breaking down the iron in much the same way that oxygen helps digest the food we eat. Classical medicine has identified a direct connection between the Stomach System and the lungs—natural therapies often treat the lungs for digestive disturbances and the stomach for lung issues like asthma.

Tissue Systems and the Digestive Cycle

The body is composed of seven main tissues systems, each of which has its own process of digestion and metabolism. Digestion is a cyclical process that

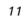

moves from one tissue system to another. From the time we begin to eat a meal, it takes between ten and fourteen days for all seven tissue systems to fully metabolize the foods. Each tissue system takes the partially processed nutrients from the system preceding it in the cycle, does its processing, and then passes the remaining nutrients to the next tissue system in the cycle to be processed further.

The first tissue system to metabolize is the *Plasma System;* this system controls the lymph and the mucous membranes of the body and is the system primarily involved in supporting the buildup of the body's cells and tissues. This system takes the digested fluids from the intestinal tract, uses the substances that it needs, and then passes the rest on to the next system, the *Blood System.* The Blood System is responsible for blood cells and the cleanliness and health of the blood. The Blood System takes the substances it needs and passes the rest on to the *Muscle System,* which governs the muscles and connective tissues. Next, the *Fat Tissue System,* controlling fat cells and tissues, receives nutrient elements from the Muscle System and passes the rest on to the *Bone Tissue System,* which is responsible for the bones. The remaining nutrients from this system move on to the *Bone and Nerve System,* governing the nerve tissues of the body. The nutrients are passed from the Bone Marrow System to the last tissue system in the cycle, the *Reproductive Organ System.* This system is the origin of the immune system and its processes and also governs the process of cell nutrition.

The Reproductive Organ System completes the most subtle aspect of nutrient metabolism. It turns the digested food into vital biological energy for the whole body. The Reproductive Organ System passes the final products of all tissue digestion to the heart, where it is returned through the circulation to the Plasma System, which is further strengthened by the full cycle so that it is able to begin the whole process over again, beginning with the next meal.

Functional disturbance in any one of these systems will compromise the health of the body and mind. The tissue systems are like links in a chain. If the Blood System is compromised, it will not be able to fulfill its role in the digestive process in an optimal way. Consequently, the Muscle System that follows in the cycle will not receive the proper nutrients, making it difficult for it to digest properly. Like dominoes falling, the other tissue systems that follow will also be affected.

Life and Digestion

Digestion and metabolism are the foundations of physical life for the body.

They are so important that in Ayurveda, the medical tradition of India, the metabolic digestive processes were named after the god Agni, meaning "fire." The term *agni* is still used today in Ayurvedic hospitals and clinics to refer to the intricate process of digestion that involves enzymes, amino acids, and digestive fluids. When the Christian Bible was translated from English into Hindi (the main language of India), the words "Holy Spirit" translated into *agni.* Ayurvedic medicine also teaches that the metabolism of digestive processes not only creates and provides nutrients for the body, but also provides the mind with its clarity, its intellectual powers of wisdom, and its ability to comprehend, create, and seek goals in life.

We need to remember that we are not what we eat but what we digest. Our growth, development, health, and well-being are determined by two main factors: the quality of the food we eat and the quality of the digestive and metabolic processes that nurture us. Food that is processed, microwaved, or is not organic is denatured (or toxic or both) and lacks the vital energies that are the foundation of our nutritional processes. In our culture, we usually eat indiscriminately for the pleasurable sensation of eating and disregard the important points of food quality, the right and wrong ways to combine and prepare foods, and the meaning of mealtimes. We seem to think that quick and easy is best, that foods should either be well salted or extra sweet and that they can be gobbled while on the run, watching TV, or driving.

Our general ignorance of the art of preparing food and the significance of nutrition has caused an almost universal health problem that has consequences for our body and mind. Some of the most popular prescription and nonprescription drugs are for chronic digestive problems including heartburn, acid reflux, colitis, irritable bowel syndrome, Crohn's disease, obesity, and high cholesterol. What additional evidence do we need that proper nutrition and digestion are key to our health?

THERAPY

CONSTIPATION

Constipation is caused by several different factors. Constipation can occur when there is insufficient fiber in the diet to provide the bulk that forms fecal material or through dehydration of the colon caused by drinking insufficient amounts of water during the day or by using diuretic medicines. Another factor that can be involved in constipation is a functional disturbance of the nerve system brought on by nervousness, stress, the inability of the body to quickly adjust to new conditions (like traveling), the use of painkillers that compromise the nerve system, and the incorrect use of enemas, colonics, laxatives, or herbs like senna, frangula, or cascara that overstimulate and fatigue the nerves of the large intestine.

Colonics and enemas, by the way, should be used only as a last resort for physically removing fecal matter from the colon in severe cases of constipation. General use of colonics and enemas negatively affect the function of the intestines. This is because the energies of the colon are "downward and outward" moving energies. Colonics and enemas reverse this energy, producing dysfunctions in the sensitive intestinal nerve systems that control bowel movements. Nonstimulating herbs and therapies like reflexology, which promote bowel movement through the natural movement of the colon system, are much healthier.

In Classical medicine, the colon is considered to control the energetic functions of the pelvic organs as well as to reflect the energies of the central nervous system. Thus, irregularities of the bowels reflect irregularities in anything that affects the organs of the pelvis, such as the kidneys, bladder, and reproductive organs. Emotional and physical stressors that affect the central nervous system also affect the functions of the colon. It is important to note that normal bowel movements should occur between 5 A.M. and 7:30 A.M. every day. If you are not having regular bowel movements during this time frame, you have constipation even though you have a bowel movement later.

If it is usual for you to have a bowel movement at another time of the day, it indicates that your "biological clock" is not functioning properly. Each one of the organ systems has a particular time in the twenty-four-hour cycle when it is most active. The active time for the large intestine is from approximately 5 A.M. to 7:30 A.M. Problems with the biological clock can be caused by functional disturbances in one or more of the other organ systems, or it may be that you have "reset" the clock to fit in with your school or work schedules. It is important not to interfere with the biological clock because it will affect all the other systems and create systemic imbalances in the body's vital processes.

It is important to regulate the bowels because the fecal matter contains toxins that are supposed to be eliminated from the body. Failure to do so results in the possibility of the colon tissues reabsorbing these toxins into the blood and spreading them throughout the body, causing chronic functional problems for other organ systems.

General Remedies

Remedy #1

- 2 teaspoons psyllium seed husks
- 1 pinch of ginger powder
- 8 ounces water
- $\frac{1}{2}$ glass fig or prune juice (if needed)
- $\frac{1}{4}$ teaspoon castor oil (if needed)

Add psyllium seed husks and ginger powder to a glass of water. Take this twice daily, making sure you also drink sufficient water throughout the day. If this mixture is not sufficient, add fig or prune juice to the psyllium-ginger water. For even stronger effect, add castor oil to the mixture.

Remedy #2

- 1 teaspoon ghee
- 8 ounces warm milk

Add ghee to a glass of warm milk at bedtime (to prepare ghee, see Remedy Preparation Techniques)

Tissue Salts

- *Kali mur.* 6X
- *Natrum phos.* 6X

Take these remedies together 3 times daily for up to one week; reduce the number of doses as symptoms begin to improve.

Spices, Herbs, and Foods

- **Artichokes**
  PREPARATION METHOD: Include in the diet
- **Asparagus**
  PREPARATION METHOD: Include in the diet
- **Chicory**
  PREPARATION METHOD: Decoction, fresh plant tincture
- **Fenugreek and flaxseed**
  PREPARATION METHOD: Pour 1 cup of boiling water over 1 teaspoon of crushed fenugreek seeds and 1 teaspoon of crushed flaxseeds. Steep 8 minutes, then drink all, including the seeds.
- **Ginger and lemon**
  PREPARATION METHOD: Mix juice of $\frac{1}{2}$ lemon with a pinch of ginger powder in a glass of water. Drink once or twice a day as needed.

Reflexology

For instructions on reflexology, see "Reflexology" under "How to Use the Therapy Section" at the beginning of Part II.

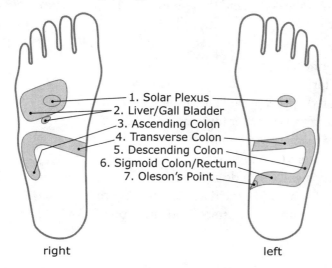

1. Solar Plexus
2. Liver/Gall Bladder
3. Ascending Colon
4. Transverse Colon
5. Descending Colon
6. Sigmoid Colon/Rectum
7. Oleson's Point

right   left

DIARRHEA

Diarrhea is caused by three main factors. One is digestive disturbance resulting from poor function of the liver, stomach, and pancreas. Another factor is overactivity of the nerve system, which involves the brain stem, vagus nerve, the nerves of the solar plexus, and/or the nerves of the small and large intestines. The third factor is irritation in the mucous membranes of the small and large intestines due to cleansing of either microbial toxins or toxins from external sources, such as chemical medicines or environmental toxins.

General Remedies

Remedy #1
- $\frac{1}{2}$ cup plain, natural yogurt
- $\frac{1}{2}$ cup of water
- $\frac{1}{8}$ teaspoon freshly grated or (a little less) powdered ginger
- $\frac{1}{8}$ teaspoon coriander
- $\frac{1}{8}$ teaspoon cinnamon

Mix the yogurt with the water. Add ginger, coriander powder, and cinnamon. If you don't have all the spices, use what you have. Eat 1–3 times per day for up to three days.

Remedy #2

- 1 small cup of prepared black coffee
- 3 teaspoons lemon juice

Mix together the coffee and the lemon juice. Drink 1–2 times per day for up to three days.

Remedy #3

- $1/2$ cup oatmeal
- 1 cup water
- $1/2$ cup cored apple, peeled and grated
- 1 pinch of ginger powder (optional)
- 1 pinch of nutmeg (optional)
- 1 pinch of cinnamon (optional)

Prepare oatmeal. (With double the usual water, it should be quite soupy.) When ready to eat, add grated apple into 1 serving of the oatmeal. If available, add ginger powder, nutmeg, and cinnamon. Take 1–3 servings daily.

Remedy #4

- $1/2$ cup rice
- 2 cups water
- 1 pinch of salt
- 1 pinch of ginger
- 1 pinch of nutmeg
- 1 pinch of cinnamon

Cook rice with a pinch of salt in 3 times as much water as usual until rice is very soft and mixture is soupy. Add a pinch each of ginger, nutmeg, and cinnamon powders. Eat one cup 1–3 times daily for up to three days.

Remedy #5

- Garlic cloves

Cut off the bottom of a garlic clove, but leave the clove in the skin. Broil clove until tender. Remove skin before eating clove. Eat 1–3 cloves several times per day.

Remedy #6

- Dried or fresh mint leaves

Make a tea (standard infusion) using the mint leaves. Steep 1 teaspoon of dried leaves or 1 tablespoon of fresh leaves in one cup of boiling water for 10 minutes. Repeat 3 times per day.

Remedy #7

- Potato

Eat 1 potato baked in its skin, per day.

Tissue Salts

For acute diarrhea in adults:

- *Ferrum phos.* 6X
- *Natrum phos.* 6X
- *Natrum sulph.* 6X
- *Kali sulph.* 6X

Take these remedies together 3 times daily for up to four days; reduce the number of doses as symptom begins to improve.

For acute diarrhea in children and infants:

- *Silicea* 6X
- *Calc. phos.* 6X
- *Natrum mur.* 6X
- *Ferrum phos.* 6X

Take these remedies together 3 times daily for up to four days; reduce the number of dosages as symptoms begin to improve.

Spices and Herbs

- **Anise seed**
  PREPARATION METHOD: Decoction, dry plant tincture
- **Basil**
  PREPARATION METHOD: Decoction, fresh plant tincture, dry plant tincture
- **Cayenne pepper**
  PREPARATION METHOD: Include in the daily diet
- **Cinnamon**
  PREPARATION METHOD: Decoction, dry plant tincture
- **Cloves**
  PREPARATION METHOD: Decoction, dry plant tincture
- **Garlic**
  PREPARATION METHOD: Fresh plant tincture
- **Ginger**
  PREPARATION METHOD: Standard hot infusion, fresh plant tincture
- **Marjoram**
  PREPARATION METHOD: Decoction, fresh plant tincture, dry plant tincture
- **Nutmeg**
  PREPARATION METHOD: Decoction, dry plant tincture
- **Turmeric**
  PREPARATION METHOD: Decoction, dry plant tincture

Foods

- **Apples**

  PREPARATION METHOD: Peel apples and boil apple peels until very soft. Eat peels and drink liquid. You also can add raw grated apple peel to oatmeal soup (oatmeal made with excess water).

- **Carrots**

  PREPARATION METHOD: Include in the diet

- **Green or black tea**

  PREPARATION METHOD: Standard hot infusion

- **Rice**

  PREPARATION METHOD: Simmer rice in a covered pan in double the amount of water usually used. Cook until rice is mushy. Strain liquid and drink, 2–3 times per day.

- **Water/salt/sugar**

  PREPARATION METHOD: Mix $1/2$ teaspoon of salt with 8 level teaspoons of sugar. Add to 1 quart of water. Drink in sips every 5 minutes throughout day and night until urine flow, which may have decreased due to dehydration, returns to normal. This mixture replaces vital substances lost during bouts of diarrhea.

Reflexology

For instructions on reflexology, see "Reflexology" under "How to Use the Therapy Section" at the beginning of Part II.

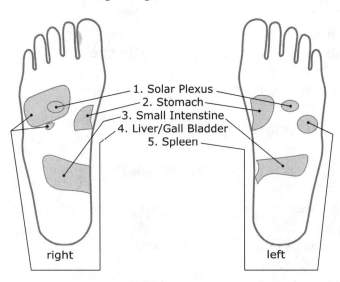

1. Solar Plexus
2. Stomach
3. Small Intenstine
4. Liver/Gall Bladder
5. Spleen

right　　　left

GAS

The formation of gas in the intestines comes from two major causes. The first is disturbances in the primary digestive system causing the improper metabolism of food and stress. Poorly metabolized nutrients form natural toxins. The second cause is exposure to chemical toxins. The lining of the intestines contains beneficial bacteria that are responsible for a major part of the digestive process. These bacteria can be harmed by environmental toxins and especially by medicines like antibiotics that cause long-term damage to the microflora of the intestines.

To help the body rebuild this microflora, take acidophilus bacteria capsules with meals for one month and eat fermented products like sauerkraut or yogurt with active cultures.

General Remedies

Remedy #1
- 1 cup of water
- Juice of $\frac{1}{2}$ lemon
- 1 pinch of baking soda

Mix together water and lemon juice with a pinch of baking soda. Drink 1–2 times daily for up to three days.

Remedy #2
- Charcoal tablets

Charcoal tablets can be purchased at most drug stores or health-food stores. Take the dosage recommended on the package.

Remedy #3
- 1 tablespoon fresh thyme, crushed, or 1 teaspoon dried thyme
- 1 cup of boiling water

Make a tea (standard infusion) by steeping thyme in boiling water. Drink 1–2 times daily for up to one week.

Remedy #4
- Juice of 1 lemon
- 1 teaspoon olive oil
- 8 ounces of water
- 1 pinch of ginger powder

Mix lemon juice and olive oil with the water. Add a pinch of ginger powder. Drink once daily.

Remedy #5

• Sauerkraut

Include in the diet daily for one week; then, include every third day for three weeks.

Tissue Salts

• *Calc. phos.* 6X
• *Natrum phos.* 6X
• *Natrum sulph.* 6X
• *Kali mur.* 6X

Take these remedies together 3 times daily for up to one week; reduce the number of doses as symptoms begin to improve.

Spices and Herbs

• **Anise seed**
  PREPARATION METHOD: Decoction, dry plant tincture
• **Black pepper**
  PREPARATION METHOD: Include in the diet
• **Caraway**
  PREPARATION METHOD: Decoction, dry plant tincture
• **Cinnamon**
  PREPARATION METHOD: Decoction, dry plant tincture
• **Garlic**
  PREPARATION METHOD: Fresh plant tincture
• **Ginger**
  PREPARATION METHOD: Standard hot infusion, fresh plant tincture
• **Marjoram**
  PREPARATION METHOD: Decoction, fresh plant tincture, dry plant tincture
• **Nutmeg**
  PREPARATION METHOD: Decoction, dry plant tincture
• **Parsley**
  PREPARATION METHOD: Decoction, fresh plant tincture, herbal wine
• **Thyme**
  PREPARATION METHOD: Decoction, fresh plant tincture, dry plant tincture

Foods

• **Celery**
  PREPARATION METHOD: Decoction

- **Lemon**
PREPARATION METHOD: Add juice from $1/2$ lemon and a pinch of ginger powder to a glass of water. Drink once or twice a day as needed.

HEMORRHOIDS

Hemorrhoids are caused by enlargement of the veins in the rectum and produce pain or discomfort around the anal opening or lower end of the rectum. This can happen when chronic constipation causes continual pressure on the blood circulation of the rectum veins or when the nerves that control the circulation are impaired by pressure blockages in the pelvis or the small of the back. A chronic disturbance in the circulation of the blood between the liver and small intestine can also cause hemorrhoids. The remedies listed below can help both digestion and circulation.

General Remedies

Remedy #1
- Aloe vera juice
Drink 2 ounces of aloe vera juice 3 times a day until symptoms improve.

Tissue Salts

- *Ferrum phos.* 6X
- *Kali phos.* 6X
- *Calc. fluor.* 6X
- *Silicea* 6X
- *Calc. phos.* 6X
Take these remedies together 3 times per day for up to one week; reduce the number of doses as symptoms begin to improve.

Spices, Herbs, and Foods

- **Artichoke**
PREPARATION METHOD: Include in the diet
- **Cabbage**
PREPARATION METHOD: Include cooked cabbage in the diet and also drink the liquid in which it was boiled
- **Castor oil**
PREPARATION METHOD: Add $1/2$ to 1 teaspoon of castor oil along with a pinch of ginger to a glass of water. Drink 1 glass per day. (Store castor oil in the refrigerator for up to one month.)

- **Fenugreek and flaxseed**

  PREPARATION METHOD: Pour 1 cup of boiling water over 1 teaspoon of crushed fenugreek seeds and 1 teaspoon of crushed flaxseeds. Steep 8 minutes, then drink all, including the seeds. (Store fenugreek and flaxseed in the refrigerator for up to one month.)

- **Lemon**

  PREPARATION METHOD: Add juice from $1/2$ lemon and a pinch of ginger powder to a glass of water. Drink once or twice a day as needed.

- **Olive oil**

  PREPARATION METHOD: Include in the diet

- **Turmeric**

  PREPARATION METHOD: Decoction, dry plant tincture

Reflexology

For instructions on reflexology, see "Reflexology" under "How to Use the Therapy Section" at the beginning of Part II.

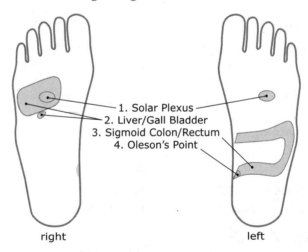

1. Solar Plexus
2. Liver/Gall Bladder
3. Sigmoid Colon/Rectum
4. Oleson's Point

right   left

PERSISTENT HICCUPS

Persistent hiccups are due to irritation of the nerve system that controls the stomach and its mucous membranes or the nerve system involved with the brain stem.

General Remedies

Remedy #1

- $1/2$ teaspoon honey

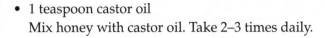

- 1 teaspoon castor oil

Mix honey with castor oil. Take 2–3 times daily.

Tissue Salts

- *Mag. phos.* 6X
- *Natrum mur.* 6X

Take these remedies together 3 times daily for up to four days; reduce the number of doses as symptoms begin to improve.

INDIGESTION AND HEARTBURN

Simple indigestion can be caused by the many factors that affect the function of the digestive system. The lining of the stomach contains small cells that produce and secrete stomach acid essential to the first stages of digestion. Heartburn can be caused by chronic disturbances in the secretion of stomach acid. Simple disturbances in this acid secretion can be caused by improper food combining, overeating, or eating at inappropriate times. If you have a tendency to heartburn, you could be tempted to take one of the many over-the-counter antacids on the market. This might bring temporary relief but in the long run it will severely compromise the stomach's functions. Stomach acid levels are regulated by chemical sensors in the lining of the stomach. These sensors turn the acid-producing cells on and off as levels rise or fall. Antacids neutralize the natural stomach acids and cause the sensors to react and switch on the acid production, setting you up for the next heartburn.

More serious and persistent problems might be caused by a small tear (hernia) in the hole (hiatus) of the diaphragm through which the intestinal nerves and the tube (esophagus) to the stomach pass. This is known as hiatal hernia, which can constrict the tube and nerves and produce constricted areas where acid can build up. The following suggestions will relieve temporary indigestion.

General Remedies

Remedy #1

- $\frac{1}{2}$ teaspoon black pepper
- $\frac{1}{2}$ teaspoon honey
- 1 pinch of ginger powder
- $\frac{1}{4}$ cup of onion juice

Mix black pepper, honey, ginger powder, and onion juice. Take 1 table-spoon directly after a meal 2 times per day for up to one week.

Remedy #2

- 1 pinch of salt
- 1 pinch of baking soda
- 1 garlic, peeled

Put a pinch of salt and a pinch of baking soda on garlic clove. Eat 1 clove per day after a meal.

Remedy #3 (for indigestion after overeating)

- Juice of $\frac{1}{2}$ lemon
- 1 pinch of baking soda
- 1 cup warm water

Add juice and a pinch of baking soda to warm water. Drink after a meal.

Remedy #4

- 1 teaspoon of anise or fennel seeds
- 1 cup hot water

Make a tea by adding the seeds to the hot water and steeping for 8 minutes. Drink 1 cup after meals 2 times per day for up to one week.

Tissue Salts

- *Natrum phos.* 6X
- *Natrum sulph.* 6X

Take these remedies together 3 times daily for up to ten days; reduce the number of dosages as symptoms begin to improve.

Spices and Herbs

- **Anise seed**

  PREPARATION METHOD: Decoction, dry plant tincture
- **Basil**

  PREPARATION METHOD: Decoction, fresh plant tincture, dry plant tincture
- **Caraway**

  PREPARATION METHOD: Decoction, dry plant tincture
- **Cardamom**

  PREPARATION METHOD: Decoction, dry plant tincture
- **Cloves**

  PREPARATION METHOD: Decoction, dry plant tincture
- **Fennel seed**

  PREPARATION METHOD: Decoction, dry plant tincture
- **Ginger**

  PREPARATION METHOD: Standard hot infusion, fresh plant tincture

Foods

- **Beets**

  PREPARATION METHOD: Include in the diet
- **Cabbage**

  PREPARATION METHOD: Include cooked cabbage in the diet and also drink liquid from cooking
- **Celery**

  PREPARATION METHOD: Decoction
- **Lemon**

  PREPARATION METHOD: Add juice from $\frac{1}{2}$ lemon and a pinch of ginger powder to a glass of water. Drink once or twice a day as needed.

Reflexology

For instructions on reflexology, see "Reflexology" under "How to Use the Therapy Section" at the beginning of Part II.

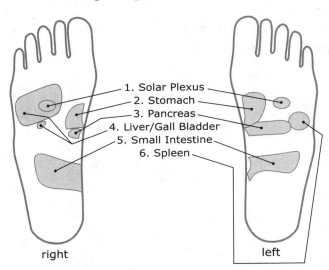

1. Solar Plexus
2. Stomach
3. Pancreas
4. Liver/Gall Bladder
5. Small Intestine
6. Spleen

right   left

VOMITING AND NAUSEA

Vomiting is one of the important ways that the body heals itself. Food that cannot be digested properly due to improper food combining or food intolerance due to allergies can influence the vomiting reflex. If the body needs to deal with an acute situation like shock, food poisoning, or other immune reactions like colds or flu, it will vomit food so as to utilize its energies in order to stabilize the main functions of the body and mind.

General Remedies

Remedy #1

- 1 dried or 1 tablespoon fresh mint
- 1 cup boiling water

Make a tea (standard infusion) by steeping mint in 1 cup of boiling water. Drink 1 cup 1–3 times daily.

Tissue Salts

- *Kali phos.* 6X
- *Natrum mur.* 6X
- *Natrum phos.* 6X
- *Natrum sulph.* 6X

Take these remedies together 3 times daily for up to three days; reduce the number of doses as symptoms begin to improve.

Reflexology

For instructions on reflexology, see "Reflexology" under "How to Use the Therapy Section" at the beginning of Part II.

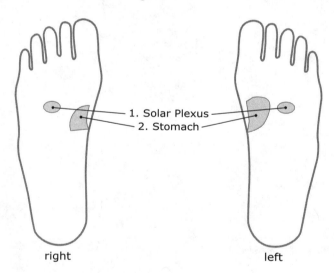

1. Solar Plexus
2. Stomach

right   left

Spices and Herbs

- **Anise seed**

    PREPARATION METHOD: Decoction, dry plant tincture

- **Basil**

    PREPARATION METHOD: Decoction, fresh plant tincture, dry plant tincture

- **Cardamom**
  PREPARATION METHOD: Decoction, dry plant tincture
- **Cinnamon**
  PREPARATION METHOD: Decoction, dry plant tincture
- **Fennel seed**
  PREPARATION METHOD: Decoction, dry plant tincture
- **Ginger**
  PREPARATION METHOD: Standard hot infusion

PARASITES AND *CANDIDA*

Parasites and *Candida* (a mycobacteria) in the digestive system are not the *causes* of problems but are the *results* of chronic dysfunctions in the nutritive tissues of the organ systems. Parasites and intestinal worms are multicelled organisms that cannot live in and are never found in a digestive system that is functioning properly. Though there are "antiparasite" and "antiworm" cures, these only address the symptoms, not the cause. The only real way of dealing with the situation is to stabilize the functions of the digestive system.

Candida is part of the way that our immune system responds to more serious functional disturbances in the digestive tract mucous membranes. These membranes are filled with millions of bacteria, called the intestinal flora, which are an essential part of the digestive process. The mucous membranes and the bacteria of the digestive system are compromised most often by toxins from nonorganic food, toxins from incomplete digestion due to chronic digestive disturbances, medicinal drugs, and toxins from mercury fillings. These toxins damage the cells of the mucous membranes. *Candida* scavenges these damaged or dying cells, removing them from the membranes and allowing new cells to develop. *Candida*, therefore, is part of the solution, it is not the problem.

Anti-*Candida* diets are not the solution. They are much too restrictive in terms of daily nourishment needed for the body and mind, and they only reduce the activity of the *Candida*; they do not alter the causes. If you have Candida, *you know that there are chronic factors affecting your digestive system and these need correcting.*

Spices and Herbs

- **Basil**
  PREPARATION METHOD: Decoction, fresh plant tincture, dry plant tincture
- **Caraway**
  PREPARATION METHOD: Decoction, dry plant tincture

- **Cinnamon**

  PREPARATION METHOD: Decoction, dry plant tincture
- **Cloves**

  PREPARATION METHOD: Decoction, dry plant tincture
- **Garlic**

  PREPARATION METHOD: Fresh plant tincture
- **Garlic and thyme**

  PREPARATION METHOD: Decoction, fresh plant tincture, dry plant tincture
- **Ginger**

  PREPARATION METHOD: Standard hot infusion, fresh plant tincture
- **Fennel seed**

  PREPARATION METHOD: Decoction, dry plant tincture
- **Lemon and ginger**

  PREPARATION METHOD: Add juice from $\frac{1}{2}$ lemon and a pinch of ginger to a glass of water. Drink once or twice a day as needed.
- **Parsley**

  PREPARATION METHOD: Decoction, fresh plant tincture, herbal wine
- **Turmeric**

  PREPARATION METHOD: Decoction, dry plant tincture

Foods

- **Apple cider vinegar**

  PREPARATION METHOD: Mix 1 teaspoon of vinegar in $\frac{1}{3}$ cup of water. Take 1–2 times daily for one week; then pause for one week and repeat the cycle for an additional week.
- **Carrots**

  PREPARATION METHOD: Include in the diet
- **Olive oil**

  PREPARATION METHOD: Include in the diet
- **Onions**

  PREPARATION METHOD: Include in the diet
- **Papaya**

  PREPARATION METHOD: Crush dried papaya seeds to a powder. Mix 3 teaspoons of powder with a glass of water. Drink 3 times per day for seven days.
- **Pumpkin seeds**

  PREPARATION METHOD: Dry plant tincture, include in the diet
- **Sauerkraut/Sauerkraut juice**

  PREPARATION METHOD: Include in the diet

GENERAL DIGESTIVE CARE

Spices and Herbs

- **Anise seed**

  THERAPEUTIC ACTION: Relieves colic, indigestion, gas, nausea, gurgling abdomen, and nervous vomiting; removes mucus

  PREPARATION METHOD: Decoction, dry plant tincture

- **Basil**

  THERAPEUTIC ACTION: Relieves indigestion, vomiting, colic, and intestinal infections

  PREPARATION METHOD: Decoction, fresh plant tincture, dry plant tincture

- **Black pepper**

  THERAPEUTIC ACTION: Relieves gas, colic, nausea, gurgling abdomen, and food poisoning

  PREPARATION METHOD: Include in the diet

- **Caraway**

  THERAPEUTIC ACTION: Relieves gas; improves digestion; antiparasitic; prevents fermentation

  PREPARATION METHOD: Decoction, dry plant tincture

- **Cardamom**

  THERAPEUTIC ACTION: Relieves gurgling abdomen, nausea, vomiting, acid reflux, and stomach pain

  PREPARATION METHOD: Decoction, dry plant tincture

- **Cayenne pepper**

  THERAPEUTIC ACTION: Restores intestinal tract; aids production of gastric juices; relieves nausea, indigestion, diarrhea, abdominal pains, and dysentery

  PREPARATION METHOD: Include in the daily diet; *not for use by children.*

- **Cinnamon**

  THERAPEUTIC ACTION: Reduces gas; antifungal, anti-*Candida,* antiparasitic; relieves nausea, chronic and acute diarrhea, chronic and acute abdominal distension, and colic; stabilizes blood sugar; relieves enteritis

  PREPARATION METHOD: Decoction, dry plant tincture

- **Chicory**

  THERAPEUTIC ACTION: Relieves vomiting, constipation, and nausea; helps liver function; relieves hepatitis

  PREPARATION METHOD: Decoction, fresh plant tincture

- **Cloves**

  THERAPEUTIC ACTION: Anti-*Candida;* antifungal; anti-inflammatory; relieves nausea, bloating, gas

PREPARATION METHOD: Decoction, dry plant tincture

- **Fennel seed**

THERAPEUTIC ACTION: Relieves painful abdomen, hiccups, nausea, vomiting, slow digestion, and colic; antifungal; fights intestinal parasites and *Candida*

PREPARATION METHOD: Decoction, dry plant tincture

- **Fenugreek seed**

THERAPEUTIC ACTION: Regulates blood sugar and balances insulin; antidiuretic; helps resolve stomach ulcers and intestinal gas; lowers cholesterol

PREPARATION METHOD: Decoction, dry plant tincture

- **Fenugreek and flaxseeds**

THERAPEUTIC ACTION: Cleanses intestinal tract

PREPARATION METHOD: Pour one cup of boiling water over 1 teaspoon of crushed fenugreek seeds and one teaspoon of crushed flaxseeds. Steep 8 minutes, then drink all, including the seeds.

- **Garlic**

THERAPEUTIC ACTION: Relieves food poisoning; reduces *Candida* and *Salmonella* infection; cleanses liver and gallbladder; promotes bile; regulates intestinal flora; relieves constipation, jaundice, intestinal colic, flatus, diarrhea, and gurgling in abdomen; reduces cholesterol

PREPARATION METHOD: Fresh plant tincture

- **Garlic and thyme**

THERAPEUTIC ACTION: Reduces intestinal fermentation; reduces flatulence and colic; relieves diarrhea; good antiparasite and antiworm medicine

PREPARATION METHOD: Decoction, fresh plant tincture, dry plant tincture

- **Ginger**

THERAPEUTIC ACTION: Supports digestion; relieves stomach ulcer, colic, nausea, loose stool, diarrhea, gas, vomiting, and food poisoning; lowers cholesterol; antifungal and antiworm therapy; relieves *Salmonella* infections

PREPARATION METHOD: Standard hot infusion, fresh plant tincture

- **Marjoram**

THERAPEUTIC ACTION: Relieves diarrhea, constipation, colic, and gurgling abdomen

PREPARATION METHOD: Decoction, fresh plant tincture, dry plant tincture

- **Nutmeg**

THERAPEUTIC ACTION: Relieves nausea, bloating, colic, and diarrhea

PREPARATION METHOD: Decoction, dry plant tincture

- **Parsley**

THERAPEUTIC ACTION: Antifungal; relieves colic, flatulence, gallstones, and jaundice

PREPARATION METHOD: Decoction, fresh plant tincture, herbal wine

- **Savory**

  THERAPEUTIC ACTION: Reduces *Candida* and other yeasts

  PREPARATION METHOD: Decoction, fresh plant tincture, dry plant tincture

- **Turmeric**

  THERAPEUTIC ACTION: Antiparasitic; relieves liver disorders and irritable bowel; protects liver; relieves gallstones; lowers cholesterol

  PREPARATION METHOD: decoction, dry plant tincture

Foods

- **Apples**

  THERAPEUTIC ACTION: Relieves diarrhea

  PREPARATION METHOD: Peel apples and boil apple peels until very soft. Eat peels and drink liquid. You also can add raw grated apple peels to oatmeal soup (oatmeal made with excess water).

- **Apple cider vinegar**

  THERAPEUTIC ACTION: Antiparasite and antiworm medicine; supports the liver's digestive functions

  PREPARATION METHOD: Mix 1 teaspoon of vinegar in $1/3$ cup water. Take 1–2 times daily for one week; then pause for one week and repeat the cycle for an additional week.

- **Asparagus**

  THERAPEUTIC ACTION: Relieves nausea, constipation and dry mouth; lowers blood sugar

  PREPARATION METHOD: Include in the diet

- **Artichoke**

  THERAPEUTIC ACTION: Reduces high cholesterol; strengthens liver/gallbladder; cleanses bowels of mucus and toxins; relieves nausea

  PREPARATION METHOD: Include in the diet

- **Beets**

  THERAPEUTIC ACTION: Aids digestion; lowers cholesterol

  PREPARATION METHOD: Include in the diet

- **Cabbage**

  THERAPEUTIC ACTION: Decongests liver; relieves heartburn

  PREPARATION METHOD: Include cooked cabbage in the diet and also drink the liquid it was cooked in.

- **Carrots**

  THERAPEUTIC ACTION: Relieves diarrhea; antiworm therapy; lowers cholesterol

  PREPARATION METHOD: Include in the diet

- **Castor oil (fresh)**

  THERAPEUTIC ACTION: Relieves constipation and intestinal tract lesions

  PREPARATION METHOD: Mix $^1/_2$ to 1 teaspoon of castor oil and a pinch of ginger powder in a glass of water. Drink once daily.

- **Castor oil pack**

  THERAPEUTIC ACTION: Relieves indigestion

  PREPARATION METHOD: Soak a piece of clean cotton cloth in fresh warm castor oil. Place on the abdomen and cover with a towel. Repeat as necessary.

- **Celery**

  THERAPEUTIC ACTION: Relieves nausea, gas, painful indigestion, and heartburn

  PREPARATION METHOD: Decoction

- **Green/black tea**

  THERAPEUTIC ACTION: Relieves diarrhea

  PREPARATION METHOD: Standard hot infusion

- **Lemon**

  THERAPEUTIC ACTION: Cleanses toxins and parasites; supports liver; relieves gastric acidity; enhances sluggish digestion; lowers cholesterol; relieves constipation, gastric acidity, heartburn, nausea, loose stool, and gas; relieves gallstones

  PREPARATION METHOD: Mix juice from $^1/_2$ lemon with a pinch of ginger powder in a glass of water. Drink once or twice a day as needed.

- **Oats**

  THERAPEUTIC ACTION: Lowers cholesterol

  PREPARATION METHOD: Include in the diet

- **Olive oil**

  THERAPEUTIC ACTION: Reduces cholesterol; antifungal and antiyeast; relieves intestinal tract lesions; relieves gallstones

  PREPARATION METHOD: Include in the diet

- **Onions**

  THERAPEUTIC ACTION: Lowers cholesterol; maintains intestinal flora; antifungal

  PREPARATION METHOD: Include in the diet

- **Papaya**

  THERAPEUTIC ACTION: Kills intestinal worms

  PREPARATION METHOD: Crush dried papaya seeds to a powder. Mix 3 teaspoons of powder with a glass of water. Drink 3 times per day for seven days.

- **Pumpkin seeds**

  THERAPEUTIC ACTION: Antiworm therapy

  PREPARATION METHOD: Dry plant tincture; include in the diet.

- **Rice**

  THERAPEUTIC ACTION: Relieves diarrhea

  PREPARATION METHOD: Simmer rice in a covered pan in double the amount of water usually used. Cook until rice is mushy. Strain liquid and drink.

- **Sauerkraut/Sauerkraut juice**

  THERAPEUTIC ACTION: Acts as probiotic; maintains intestinal flora

  PREPARATION METHOD: Include in the diet

General Cleanse for Intestinal Tract

Blend 1 part raw spinach and 1 part apple juice in a blender. Drink 1–2 glasses daily; if available, 1 hour after drinking above mixture, drink 1 cup of celery juice followed an hour later by 1 cup of carrot juice.

General Liver Cleanse

Mix juice of $\frac{1}{2}$ lemon with 1 teaspoon of olive oil and $\frac{1}{8}$ teaspoon of ginger powder in a glass of water. Drink daily.

Reflexology

For instructions on reflexology, see "Reflexology" under "How to Use the Therapy Section" at the beginning of Part II.

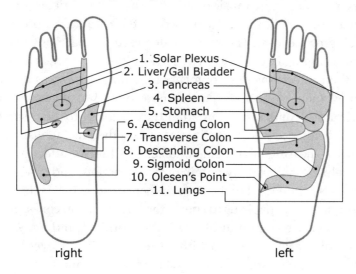

1. Solar Plexus
2. Liver/Gall Bladder
3. Pancreas
4. Spleen
5. Stomach
6. Ascending Colon
7. Transverse Colon
8. Descending Colon
9. Sigmoid Colon
10. Olesen's Point
11. Lungs

right   left

EAR AILMENTS

TEACHING

If you recall, during gestation the cells of our tissues and organs develop from one of three original embryological tissue systems. The endoderm produces cells that develop into the digestive tract, while the mesoderm produces cells that develop into bones, muscles, kidneys, and reproductive organs. The third system, the ectoderm, produces cells that develop into our nerve tissues. It is out of this last system that the ear develops. Because the tissues and organs within each system originate from the same group of cells, they remain connected, particularly in function. This means that the ear plays an active role in the development of all nerve tissues, including those in the brain.

Research has shown that when sound stimulates our ears, certain pathways in the brain are also stimulated and, as a result, support the nerve tissues responsible for coordinating how our bodies move. This formation occurs primarily in the first twelve years of childhood, though it remains active throughout one's entire life. The stimulation of sound helps many areas of the brain develop. Infants and young children exposed to the rhythms and harmonies in good quality music or nursery rhymes experience greater brain development than children not exposed to these sounds. Soft music or a mother's singing has been proven to create peace and harmony in the senses of a child developing in utero, even as early as the fourth week of pregnancy.

Sound, then, affects the development of the mind as well as the coordination and movement of the body. Furthermore, our sense of hearing orients us to our environment and, just as importantly, contributes to the tissue-building processes and enhances their functions as well as their metabolism. In fact, all of our senses—hearing, sight, smell, taste, and touch—affect our physical body and help create harmony within our cells, organs, and tissues.

The ear is also connected to the development of speech. It is the silent partner of the organs that enable us to speak: the tongue, vocal cords, and mouth. Through the ear, we communicate with the world around us. We "see" as much with our hearing as we do with our eyes. While the eyes see physical objects, the ear sees the spaces within which we move and live. This concept is important to understand because our sense of security, of being at home in our world, is partly based on listening to the world. Just think how suddenly insecure and out of balance we feel when our ears become plugged due to a head cold or riding in an airplane or swimming under water. Space is the "womb" of all creation—all things, from atoms to cells, form and grow in space. Our ear is the organ that relates to this space and makes it possible for our body to sense what it cannot see visually.

The ear is designed to ground and balance us. In the inner ear, tiny nerve fibers float in a small chamber of fluid. The fluid moves the nerve fibers, which in turn send signals to our brain. As we move, this fluid moves like the bubble in a carpenter's level. When our inner ear nerve system functions properly, the fluid moves properly, stimulating the nerves, and we experience a sense of balance and gravity, which affects our psychological well-being just as it does our bodies. Any condition that interferes with the inner ear's function can have both physical *and* psychological effects. When our sense of balance is affected even a little, we feel emotionally insecure or ungrounded. We become disoriented in space and physically we may feel dizzy and disoriented.

In the Bible, the original word for "ear" and "hearing"—*ozen*—meant equilibrium or stability of the mind and body. If chronic problems interfere with the function of the ear, one subtle emotional symptom may be a feeling of uneasiness with life in general. This feeling may be more noticeable during times of quiet and rest. The lack of this basic stability can sometimes be seen in children who are labeled hyperactive and restless, who constantly change positions, talk too loud, and generally show signs of being uneasy. These symptoms are often due to chronic ear problems that were never completely resolved.

The functions of the ear and our hearing are also connected to the functions of the liver and gallbladder, the kidney, the inner throat, and the upper respiratory tract. Traditional Chinese medicine recognizes and works with these connections as a foundation for any kind of therapy involving the ear. When these organs function well, we hear better. This concept may sound rather strange to us, but it has been an integral part of Classical medical practice for hundreds of years and has enabled practitioners to recognize disease patterns and assist the body in regaining balance and harmony through proper therapies.

THERAPY

EAR INFLAMMATION

Tissue Salts

First Stage of Ear Inflammation:
Look for any or all of these symptoms: clear mucus; throbbing, sharp, stitching, radiating pains; tension and feeling of burning and fullness in affected area of the ear.

- *Ferrum phos.* 6X

On the first day, give 1 dose every $\frac{1}{2}$ hour (except when sleeping) until any of the symptoms begin to change. When any of the original symptoms improve, reduce the dosage to every 2 hours for one day, then to 3 times daily for three additional days. If symptoms change, for example, from the first stage of inflammation to the second stage, then start using the remedies that match the symptoms listed below. For adults, 1 dose equals 4 tablets; for children under ten, 1 dose is 2 tablets.

Remember, especially if you have small children, the first indications of an immune response, no matter where or why, are changes in "normal" behavior. Loss of appetite, or being fussy with food, unusual irritability, restlessness, excessive tiredness, or dissatisfaction with play and toys that usually gratify indicate an imbalance. This is the time to respond by giving rest, cutting down on foods, observing carefully, being patient, and, if possible, starting with gentle but effective treatments such as chamomile tea or, as suggested above, *Ferrum phos.* 6X.

Second Stage of Ear Inflammation:

Any or all of these symptoms may be present: earache; whitish mucus; swollen glands; stuffy sensation in ear along with "deafness"; cracking noise when swallowing, chewing, or blowing nose.

- *Kali mur.* 6X
- *Calc. phos.* 6X
- *Ferrum phos.* 6X (if fever is present)

Take these remedies together as directed above.

Third Stage of Ear Inflammation:

Look for any or all of these symptoms: earache; yellowish or greenish mucus; pus coming from the ear.

- *Kali sulph.* 6X
- *Natrum sulph.* 6X
- *Silicea* 6X
- *Kali phos.* 6X

Take these remedies together as directed above.

Healing After Ear Inflammation:

The following remedies will help support the healing process during convalescence after symptoms have been resolved.

- *Kali phos.* 6X
- *Calc. phos.* 6X

Take these remedies together twice a day for four days.

GENERAL CARE REGARDLESS OF EAR SYMPTOMS

General Remedies

Remedy #1

- ¼ teaspoon fennel seeds (if readily available; if not, make the tea without fennel)
- 1 cup water
- 15 dried chamomile buds (available in health food stores), or chamomile tea bags
- ½ teaspoon raw cane sugar (turbinado sugar)

Chamomile helps reduce fever, calms and soothes nerves, and supports digestion. Fennel reduces heat and balances all body processes. For 1 cup of this tea, simmer the fennel seeds for 5 minutes in water, then turn off the heat and add the chamomile buds or chamomile tea bag. For infants, use 8 chamomile buds per cup; for children age one and older and for adults, use 15 buds per cup. Let the tea steep, covered, for 10 minutes. Take 3 doses per day.

Adult dose is 1 cup. Dosage for children younger than two years, ½ to 1 teaspoon; two to four years, 2 teaspoons; four to seven years, 1 tablespoon; seven to eleven years, 2 tablespoons. You can adjust doses for the size of the child.

Herbs and Spices

- **Fennel (powdered)**
  THERAPEUTIC ACTION: reduces heat and balances all functions in the body
- **Coriander (powdered)**
  THERAPEUTIC ACTION: reduces the effects of heat and inflammation
- **Peppermint (leaf)**
  THERAPEUTIC ACTION: antibiotic, cools inflammation, and soothes nerves
- **Ginger (powder)**
  THERAPEUTIC ACTION: supports the mucous membranes and harmonizes all the body's processes
- **Marjoram**
  THERAPEUTIC ACTION: expels mucus, helps the body clear toxins, and supports the immune system
- **Thyme**
  THERAPEUTIC ACTION: antibiotic, clears mucous membranes, and helps detox tissues
- **Cumin**
  THERAPEUTIC ACTION: heals tissues, soothes nerves, and balances metabolism

To make spice and herbal teas: Steep 1 teaspoon of dried spice or herb in

1 cup of water. For fresh herbs, double the amount of herb. For children under age twelve, use half the amount of spices or herbs. Pour boiling water over the spice or herb and let steep, covered, for 10–20 minutes. Pour the infused tea through a strainer before drinking.

Adult dose is 1 cup. Dosage for children younger than 2 years, $\frac{1}{2}$ to 1 teaspoon; 2–4 years, 2 teaspoons; 4–7 years, 1 tablespoon; 7–11 years, 2 tablespoons. You can adjust doses for the size of the child.

Foods

These foods will help the healing process:

- Apple (grated or juice)
- Avocado
- Broccoli (lightly steamed)
- Cabbage (lightly boiled)
- Carrot juice or grated carrot, with every meal, if possible
- Cranberries (medium cooked or pure juice
- Green pepper (cooked or stir-fried)
- Honey
- Kale (steamed, medium boiled, or stir-fried)
- Lettuce
- Olive oil
- Onions (boiled, baked, or stir-fried)
- Orange juice
- Parsley, raw or lightly boiled, with every meal, if possible
- Pineapple juice
- Potato (mashed)
- Radishes
- Red grapes (fruit or juice)
- Rice (boiled well)
- Spinach (steamed or stir-fried)
- Unprocessed cane sugar (only a little) diluted with water

Regardless of the symptoms, avoid the following foods:

- Caffeine
- Corn oil
- Dairy products
- Eggs
- Foods containing additives and preservatives such as MSG, food dyes, and artificial flavors
- Meat
- Oats
- Partially hydrogenated oils
- Peanuts
- Processed sugars
- Safflower oil
- Soy products
- Sunflower oil
- Wheat products

GENERAL CARE FOR FEVER DURING EAR INFLAMMATION

See the entry "Fever" on page 164.

Tissue Salts

For all fevers:
- *Ferrum phos.* 6X

If fever rises at night, add:
- *Kali sulph.* 6X

If fever is high and accompanied by weakness and exhaustion, add:
- *Kali phos.* 6X
- *Calc. phos.* 6X

Take the remedies every 30 minutes up to 8 times on the first day. For the next two days, take appropriate remedies 4–6 times per day. Reduce the number of doses as symptoms begin to improve.

GENERAL CARE FOR THE FOLLOWING EAR SYMPTOMS:

⊛ **Pain**

⊛ **Feeling of fullness with sharp or stabbing pains**

⊛ **Painful pressure behind the eardrum**

⊛ **Fluid or pus coming from the ear**

The above symptoms may indicate an acute inflammation of the middle ear, the inner ear, or the Eustachian tubes. When there is an acute immune process going on in the ear, we often experience a feeling of fullness and a sharp or stabbing pain deep in the ear behind the eardrum. This occurs due to swelling caused by an increase in the fluids surrounding the inner ear tissues. The swelling presses on the nerves in the sensitive tissues of the ear and we feel pain. This extra fluid is composed of toxins, such as destroyed bacteria, that are being transported away from the tissues; immune substances, like white blood cells, that help restore health to the tissues; and nutrients to help rebuild and nourish all the cells and the tissues in the area.

Inflammation and infections are not really diseases, but indicate that the immune system is attempting to restore a healthy balance to the body's tissues. The immune system works in stages, each representing a step in the way that the body attempts to heal itself. The body is a magnificent organism, which communicates with us through symptoms. If we observe this language of symptoms carefully, we can learn what our bodies are doing to achieve health and balance. Different stages of the immune process produce different symptoms. Each symptom reveals a scenario that we can respond to with appropriate treatments.

When the mucous membranes of the ear are inflamed, it tells us that the immune system is doing the job it is meant to do. Despite our discomfort, inflammation actually helps the body cleanse itself of old microbes and toxins that impede tissue function. The extra fluid causing the inflammation is actually a healing mechanism.

Everyone experiences inflammation of mucous membranes at one time or another; it is a sign of a healthy body. From infancy to the age of puberty, it is natural for children to have very active mucous membranes, which often have more periods of inflammation than are usual for adults. This is due to the maturing and development of the immune system and is one of the ways that the body adjusts to its environment. Chronic ear infections may occur when the original immune response is impaired and fails to heal completely. Perhaps antibiotics were used repeatedly or vaccines affected the immune system so that it could not complete the healing process, or perhaps toxins released from chemicals in medicines, nonorganic foods, municipal drinking water, or mercury fillings interfered with healing. Chronic emotional stress can also trigger inflammatory immune responses.

General Remedies

Remedy #1
- Cover the neck with a scarf to keep cold air and drafts away. Remove only if there is fever.

Remedy #2
- 1 garlic clove
- 2 tablespoons olive oil
- $\frac{1}{8}$ teaspoon pure cane sugar (turbinado sugar) or raw honey
- $\frac{1}{8}$ teaspoon coriander powder (if available)

Garlic is a very powerful antibiotic, antiviral, and antifungal. It cleanses tissues of all toxins and strengthens the immune system. Olive oil decreases the heat in mucous membranes, calms the nerves, and supports metabolic processes. Cane sugar decreases heat in mucous membranes, soothes the nerves, and is antiseptic. Raw unboiled honey cuts mucus buildup, helps resolve inflammation, and contains immune substances. Coriander helps absorption, reduces heat, and detoxes tissues.

For adults and children age two and older: Crush garlic clove into olive oil.

Mix in pure cane sugar (if not available, use honey or nothing at all) and coriander powder. Let the mixture sit for 2–3 hours (up to 12 hours if the situation is not acute). Soak a small piece of cotton or a cotton ball in the oil. **When using with children ages two to five, remove any garlic pieces that cling to the cotton.** Form the cotton to fit in the ear and then gently insert it just far enough so it stays in place by itself. Insert another cotton ball soaked in the oil mixture into the other ear, even if it is does not hurt, because this supports the full healing function occurring in the ears.

Change the cotton after 4 hours. Cotton soaked in oil and garlic can remain in both ears throughout the night. This mixture will be fresh for one week when refrigerated.

For children under age two: Use only olive oil on the cotton ball. Remove the cotton piece after 1 hour, and wait 30 minutes before reinserting a fresh cotton ball soaked in olive oil. Repeat. Do not leave in the ear overnight. Rather, at night very gently apply oil with a cotton swab just to the front part of the ear canal, never going in deep with the cotton swab, and insert a clean piece of cotton dipped in a little olive oil in the ear before sleep. Put a piece of cotton dipped in a small amount of oil in *both* ears, even the one that is not hurting, in order to support the full healing function in the ears.

Note: Do not take garlic tablets or raw garlic internally when there is inflammation or fever. If the eardrum has ruptured due to a buildup of pus, you will see drainage of fluid or pus from the ear. This is not an emergency situation. The eardrum is made to rupture in order to protect the sensitive inner tissues of the ear by releasing fluids or pus. If this occurs, put a few drops of the oil mixture on a piece of cotton and place it in the ear, as directed above. However, *do not use the drops directly in the ear.* If you are in doubt, consult your doctor or natural health-care professional.

Remedy #3
- 2 tablespoons olive oil
- 6 drops fresh garlic oil
- 6 drops onion juice
- $\frac{1}{8}$ teaspoon coriander

Prepare oil mixture as described above in #2, but add 2 drops of onion juice per 1 teaspoon of oil. Onion cleanses the mucous membranes, increases immunity, and gives strength to the body. If you finely grate an onion or blend it in a food processor, juice will form. Gently rub the mixture underneath the ear lobe, around the bone in back of the ear, as well as over the entire ear. Repeat several times throughout the day. You can do this treatment in addition to #2.

Note: Do not take garlic tablets or raw garlic internally when there is inflammation or fever.

Remedy #4
- Fresh ginger
- Sesame oil

Another good oil mixture involves combining one drop of juice from grated fresh ginger with two drops of sesame oil. Put the oil mixture on a cotton ball and place it in the ear as described above. This can be alternated with the garlic oil mixture in #2.

Ginger is called "the King of Herbs" in Tibetan medicine. It supports the mucous membranes and harmonizes all of the body's processes. Sesame oil soothes the nerves, nurtures and builds all tissues, and supports all healing processes.

Remedy #5
- Ear drops containing mullein and garlic (available at most health food stores)

Mullein is anti-inflammatory, supports the mucous membranes, and soothes the nerves. You can alternate this oil with the garlic oil mixture described in #2 every 12 hours. Heat the bottle containing the oil in a pan of warm water so that the oil becomes lukewarm. Use 8 drops for an adult, 5 drops for children between ages one and five, and 2 drops for infants. Insert a small piece of cotton into the ear after administering the drops. Do not use this method if the eardrum has ruptured.

Note: Do not take garlic tablets or raw garlic internally when there is inflammation or fever.

Remedy #6
- 1 thin slice onion
- 1 garlic clove (for children under two, omit the garlic)
- Several inner leaves of white or green cabbage

A very good way to abet the healing process and encourage the drainage of tissues that have been working hard to heal an infection is to make a simple compress. Onion, garlic, and cabbage purify the blood, draw out toxins, and heal tissues. Place onion, garlic, and cabbage in a blender or food processor, or chop finely by hand, making sure to save the juices. Purée the ingredients into porridge consistency. Place the puréed mixture in the center of a clean piece of cotton, such as a dish towel, and trifold the cloth so that the mixture won't fall out. Place this compress just beneath and behind the ear.

With small children, hold the compress in place with a cap that goes down over the ears. Leave the compress on for up to 1 hour or until the skin under the compress turns slightly red. Then make a fresh compress using only puréed cabbage leaves and set in place behind the ear for an additional hour. This can be done several times per day.

Remedy #7

- 1 teaspoon sea salt or regular salt
- 1 cup hot water

Salt counteracts toxins, purifies tissues, and reduces inflammation. Make ear drops by dissolving sea salt or regular salt in hot water. When the mixture cools to room temperature, use an eyedropper or soak up the solution on a piece of cotton and place 5–6 drops into the ear. Place a small dry piece of cotton or cotton ball in the ear after administering the drops. You can do this several times a day. Do not use this method if the eardrum has ruptured.

Tissue Salts

Refer to the section on ear inflammation for recommended tissue salts.

GENERAL CARE FOR THE FOLLOWING EAR SYMPTOMS:

❀ **Discomfort but no sharp pain**

❀ **Plugged-up feeling with itching and pressure in the ear canal near the eardrum**

❀ **Discomfort worsens or becomes better when you pull on the ear lobe**

The discomfort could be due to a buildup of wax in the ear. Earwax is a natural substance secreted by the tissues in the ear canal to protect the canal and the eardrum. Many of the body's secretions, like earwax, phlegm, and tears, have a dual purpose: they are part of tissue-cleansing processes and also protect and rejuvenate important external organs like the eyes, ears, nose, and skin. The purpose of earwax is to keep the skin of the ear canal resilient and sensitive to sound and to prevent small particles like dust from settling in the eardrum. For the most part, the wax cleanses itself within the ear canal, unnoticed by us. In some cases, though, the earwax builds up, creating pressure or pain in the ear canal and even inhibiting hearing. Small insects or other objects can also enter the ear canal unnoticed and produce the same symptoms.

If you are in doubt about the cause of symptoms, consult your doctor or natural health-care professional. Do not attempt to clean the ear with a cotton swab or other object inserted into the ear.

General Remedy

- 2–3 drops of almond oil or liquid glycerin

Almond oil is soothing to the nerves, reduces mucus, and strengthens tissues. Glycerin builds up tissues, strengthens nerves, and dissolves hardened deposits. Lay the head on one side. Using an eyedropper, slowly put drops of either almond oil or liquid glycerin (available at pharmacies) into the ear. Let it flow deep into the ear. Do the same with the other ear. The oil will run out when you stand up, leaving enough in the ear to soften the wax. On the following day, again using the eyedropper, put 3–4 drops of lukewarm water into the ear, then let it circulate and run out again. Do this for two days. Adults can use a rubber ear syringe to rinse out the ear. Use light pressure on the syringe and repeat the next day, if necessary. If the problem persists, see your doctor or natural healthcare professional for an ear examination.

TREATMENT FOR THE FOLLOWING EAR SYMPTOMS:

- **Cold symptoms are present and hearing is difficult**

- **Blocked-up feeling making it hard to hear**

- **Itching, irritating feeling that seems to extend from your ear down the inside of your jaw and into the back of your throat and which may disappear when you swallow**

- **Ear occasionally "pops," allowing you to hear better**

- **When you speak, the sound seems as if it comes from inside your head**

A cold or flu can cause the mucous membranes in the ear to swell, creating a temporary blockage in the eustachian tube. The mucous membranes of the upper respiratory tract (nose, sinuses, ears, throat, and eustachian tubes) are all connected with one another. The eustachian tube acts like a vent that opens into the throat on one end and extends into the middle ear on the other end. It helps the middle ear drain naturally, even when mucous membranes are inflamed, so that pressures don't build up inside the ear. It also allows air to move in and out of the middle ear, thereby equalizing the air pressure between the inside of the ear and the outside air.

When the mucous membranes of the eustachian tubes are irritated and swell, this blocks the free passage of air and fluids passing from the middle ear through the tubes into the mouth. As a result, you may feel "plugged up" and may not be able to hear as well. If this is the case, your ear may pop when you swallow, allowing you to hear better. The "pop" occurs when the eustachian tube reopens.

General Remedy

- 1 cup of water
- 1 teaspoon sea salt (or table salt)
- 1 tablespoon liquid glycerin (if available)

Use these ingredients to make nose drops, which can help open up the passages of the eustachian tubes. Salt counteracts toxins, purifies tissues, and reduces inflammation. Glycerin builds up tissues, strengthens nerves, and dissolves hardened deposits.

Boil water, let it cool to warm, and add salt (preferably sea salt but use what you have) and liquid glycerin (if you have it). Let the water cool to lukewarm. Place 10 drops of liquid into each nostril with the head held back so the drops can go through the entire nasal passage. Repeat this several times a day.

Tissue Salts

- *Kali mur.* 6X

Take this remedy every 45 minutes up to 6 times a day.

If this does not relieve the congestion, add:

- *Kali sulph.* 6X
- *Silicea* 6X

Take all three remedies together 4–5 times daily for up to two days. Reduce the number of doses as symptoms begin to improve.

Foods

Avoid sugars and sweets, dairy products, and wheat products as long as symptoms persist.

RED, SORE OUTER EAR OR EAR LOBE

These symptoms could indicate an insect bite or bruising from pressure or trauma on the outer ear. It could also be the beginning of a small pimple forming in the skin of the ear. The job of the outer ear is to work like a living funnel, helping channel sound to our eardrum. The outer ear also has nerves that directly affect hearing itself. We hear with the outer ear as well as the eardrum and the tissues inside the ear.

The outer ear is very sensitive, being mostly cartilage, blood vessels, and nerves. Because of this, it can bruise easily. Insect bites, sleeping in an awkward position, or even an earring can produce redness, swelling, and irritation. In addition, the surface of our outer ear has many reflex points that relate to different organs and functions of the body. We can see these points if we look at a chart of acupuncture points (see below). If there is any chronic disturbance of an organ system, the reflex point on the ear connected to this organ can act up, producing symptoms like swelling or a small pimple.

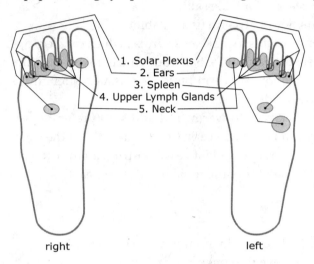

1. Solar Plexus
2. Ears
3. Spleen
4. Upper Lymph Glands
5. Neck

right   left

General Remedies

Remedy #1

Do not wear earrings until all symptoms have been gone for at least a week. You may be reacting to the metals used in the earrings as well as irritation from the earring itself.

Remedy #2

• 1 teaspoon chamomile buds or 1 chamomile tea bag per cup

Make chamomile tea, using chamomile flower buds or chamomile tea bag. Soak a piece of cotton or cotton cloth in the lukewarm tea. Apply to the outer ear for 1 hour.

Remedy #3

• Castor oil (fresh) or almond oil

Apply castor or almond oil to the outer ear 2–3 times daily. Castor oil improves tissue metabolism and the building of tissues; it is very good for drawing out toxins, dissolving cysts, and resolving tumors.

Remedy #4

• Mullein and garlic oil

Health food stores usually carry ear oil containing mullein and garlic. Apply the oil to the outer ear 2–3 times daily.

Tissue Salts

- *Silicea* 6X

Take the remedy 4–5 times daily. After two days, reduce the number of doses to 2–3 times per day for up to fourteen days.

PAIN IN JAW, GUMS, OR TEETH WITH DISCOMFORT IN THE EAR

These symptoms could indicate that the pain in the ear is a reflex from tooth or gum diseases. The eustachian tube reaches from the middle ear to an opening in the back of the throat. Because of this, chronic infections in the mouth, including problems with teeth such as cavities, micro-infections in the roots of the teeth, root canals, mercury fillings, gum disease, and teething in infants, can irritate the eustachian tube and be felt in the ear.

Also, nerve reflexes from the teeth and gums can influence the ear. Mercury fillings release a vapor of mercury ions that produces irritation and creates low-grade infections of the mucous membranes in the mouth. If you have a combination of two or more metals in the mouth, such as mercury and gold, a slight galvanic electrical current will be produced, causing functional problems that will influence the mucous membranes and the digestive system. Root canals can produce chronic micro-infections that you can't feel in the roots of the tooth; these bacteria can affect the mucous membranes of the throat and ear, as well as the sinuses.

Another possible cause of these symptoms is chronic tension in the joint of the jaw itself. This large joint, the temporomandibular joint (TMJ), can be chronically tense, causing reflexes to the ear and eustachian tubes that can affect your hearing. This is what happens when you grit your teeth or grind your teeth, which causes tension in the jaw muscles. Have a good dentist check your teeth and gums for any problems.

General Remedies

Remedy #1
- Nonfluoride toothpaste
- 10 drops Lady's Mantle tincture
- 10 drops vinegar
- 1 pinch of sea salt (or other salt)

Brush teeth with the nonfluoride toothpaste. Rinse your mouth for at least 1 minute after each brushing with Lady's Mantle tincture (available at health food stores), vinegar, and salt, all dissolved in a shot glass of water. Lady's Mantle stops inflammation, nourishes tissues, and heals wounds.

Remedy #2

- 1 tablespoon sunflower oil (organic)

Sunflower oil cools inflammation, detoxes tissues, and reduces mucus. This treatment cleanses the entire mouth of all toxins, heavy metals, and unwanted microbes. In the morning before eating or brushing the teeth, swish 1 tablespoon of organic sunflower oil in the mouth for 10 minutes or until it gets somewhat frothy. It will be whitish and is filled with toxins. Spit out the fluid—be careful not to swallow any of it. Then rinse your mouth with water and brush your teeth again. Remember, the tissues in the mouth are an extension of the tissues in the stomach and intestines. Our digestion has a great influence on all mucous membranes in the mouth.

If you feel you have chronically tense jaw muscles from stress, try getting in the habit of noticing this tension and then releasing it by keeping the teeth slightly parted and relaxing the jaw. Then exercise the jaw muscles by opening the mouth wide, but not so wide as to hurt the muscles, and moving the jaw from side to side for a minute several times per day.

Tissue Salts

To relieve muscle tension in the jaw:

- *Mag. phos.* 6X
- *Calc. phos.* 6X

Take these remedies together 3 times per day for seven to ten days. Reduce the number of doses as symptoms begin to improve.

PAIN AFTER SWIMMING OR FLYING IN A PLANE

This symptom indicates a slight congestion of the eustachian tubes when they are subjected to air pressure changes. In order to function correctly, the inner air pressure of the middle ear must be the same as the air pressure of the outside air. When we are traveling on an airplane or swimming more than 3 feet underwater, the outer air pressure changes. If the eustachian tube is slightly congested, a feeling of pressure will develop in the ear due to this difference in air pressures.

General Remedies

Remedy #1

Try yawning and opening the mouth wide, then moving it from side to side to open the eustachian tubes. Or chew on a piece of cotton just as if you were chewing gum.

Remedy #2

- 1 teaspoon sea salt or table salt
- 1 cup warm water

Mix 1 teaspoon of sea salt with 1 cup of warm water and stir until the salt dissolves. Gargle the mixture in the back of your throat several times a day.

Tissue Salts

- *Kali mur.* 6X

Take 3 doses a day for three days before flying (or swimming) and 1 dose every 2 hours while flying.

Foods

Avoid sugars and sweets, dairy products, and wheat products as long as symptoms last.

Reflexology

For instructions on reflexology, see "Reflexology" under "How to Use the Therapy Section" at the beginning of Part II.

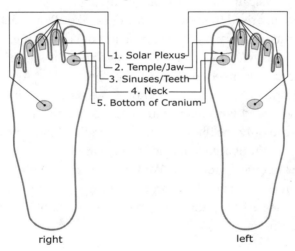

right   left

GENERAL HEALTH OF THE EAR

Boil a small washcloth or other cotton material for 5 minutes. Fold one corner into a small tight tube. Bite down firmly on this with the back molars for 1 minute. Repeat 2 more times. This stimulates the reflexes to the ear and to the roots of the teeth. You can also use a cotton tampon for this purpose, like the ones that dentists use when working on teeth. This can be done 1–2 times daily as part of your general health regime.

EYE AND VISION PROBLEMS

TEACHING

Our eyes allow us to see things by bringing us into contact with, and making us part of, the environment that we share with all other things. Seeing gives us a sense of having a relationship and an impact on everything around us. The sense of sight also helps develop our identity. It imparts the sense of being alive in a world filled with other beings who have their own identities.

The eyes do not just see objects but lead the living energies of light from the outer world into the inner world of our body and mind. Bringing the outer world into the functions of our inner world creates new life and is known as metabolism, a Greek word meaning "the transformation of matter." When we use the word *metabolism,* we usually refer to our digestion processes. Digestion involves transforming the nutrients from foods and liquids into the tissues and energies of the body, thereby enabling us to form and maintain our identities, both physically and psychologically.

You might be surprised to know that the eyes, like all our sense organs, are involved with this primary metabolic function of supporting, building, and nourishing our lives. We can say that our eyes digest the spectrums of energy in light, just as the stomach and intestines digest food. As odd as it may sound, this digestion of color and light nourishes us physically and emotionally. Color is associated with particular qualities of light. We can't see colors in the dark; we can only see them when the energy of light reveals them. One of the most important qualities of color is its heating and cooling properties, which affect all biological processes. We speak of cooling colors and warming colors. Digestion is a heat and light process; the eye with its ability to see and mediate visual images brings the energies of heat and light found in color into our metabolic systems.

How the Eye Sees Color

When we look at something, we are able to see it because light passes into the deep interior of our eyes and reflects onto the back wall of tissue called the retina. The retina contains a light-sensitive pigment. When light strikes this color-sensing pigment, it is "digested" and metabolized, producing biochemical substances that affect the tissues of the optic nerve. These substances stimulate the part of the brain that re-creates an image in our nerve system. Thus, before we even "see" an object, we begin to digest it. Such visual digestion doesn't just affect the nerves of the brain centers but carries the light and heat energies found in the color of matter to all of the body's tissue systems, enabling them to metabolize and function properly. The metabolic energies of heat and light are carried through the body by the Liver/Gallbladder System, which controls the various parts of the eye's tissues. Because of this connection between the liver and the eye, it is important for our vision that the liver function well. Diseases of the eye and vision problems are often caused by long-term functional disturbances in the liver and gallbladder.

Color affects our well-being: certain colors make us feel more at peace and turn us inward to quietness, while other colors stimulate us toward more outward activities. It would be very hard, for instance, to sleep well in a room painted fire-engine red! The color red is a hot, active, dynamic, and stimulating color that increases our activity. Shades of blue, on the other hand, are more cooling, peaceful, and restful colors, much more suitable for inducing sleep.

Seeing and the Psyche

Seeing not only stimulates our digestive metabolism but also plays a crucial role in our psyche and the responses of our consciousness. Our vision is truly "visionary" in that it helps us to comprehend and understand things, making the digestion occurring in our eyes an important part of our consciousness. We often say, "I see!" when we mean that we have understood something. Seeing is not just a matter of observing objects as they appear in the space around us, but of really comprehending and understanding their *meaning*. The eyes provide our minds with "digested vision," with ways of understanding and comprehending life. The functions of seeing are also directly connected to our creativity, enabling us to discover new meanings and relationships within the space of our environment or the formation of our thoughts. This is the true meaning of vision.

The Embryological Development of the Eye

In the embryo, the different tissues of the eye develop from the mesoderm and the ectoderm. These embryological tissues are the same ones that create the brain, nerves, heart, lungs, and reproductive organs. We can say that the eye and its vision help harmonize the heart and the nervous system and bring us into a deep creative relationship with the world around us.

A clear membrane called the conjunctiva covers the outer part of the eye. It protects the sensitive tissues of the eyeball, while at the same time allowing light in. The tissue of this membrane also supplies nutrients and provides fluid to the eyeball to keep it moist. Furthermore, the conjunctiva tissues have cells that relate to the nerves, making them very sensitive to anything entering the eye that might be harmful. The eye's membranes and those of the upper respiratory tract are connected to one another in a seamless system. The conjunctiva can therefore be compromised by a cold, allergic reactions, problems with gums or teeth, or sinus problems. When inflamed or irritated, the conjunctiva can produce a slight burning sensation, a feeling of stickiness around the eyelids, a stinging and irritated feeling when the eye is open, or the sensation of sandy grit rubbing against the eye when blinking.

THERAPY

EYE INJURIES OR IRRITANTS IN EYE

If anything has gotten into your eye, like dust or an eyelash, the eye will produce tears to wash it away. Often this action is enough. But if the irritant is something like sand or grit, even though the tears may have washed it out, the sand or grit may have scratched the outer membrane of the eyeball.

General Remedies

Remedy #1
- 10 chamomile buds, or 1 chamomile tea bag
- $\frac{1}{4}$ teaspoon salt

Prepare an eyewash by making a cup of chamomile tea: steep chamomile buds or chamomile tea bag in hot water for 15 minutes. Add salt to the tea. When the solution has cooled to lukewarm, pour it into an eyecup or shot glass. Put your eye down over the glass, press the glass against your face, and lift your head. Keep the eye open while the solution bathes the eye. Do this several times a day. If you have aloe vera gel or liquid, you can also gently rub this around the area of the eye several times a day.

If you have injured your eye, or pain persists for more than 30 minutes, contact your physician immediately. Then cover the eye completely with a piece of cotton soaked (not dripping!) in chamomile tea until the doctor can be seen.

EYES THAT STING, ITCH, ARE RED, OR FEEL STICKY/GRITTY

This is a sign of inflammation of the outer membrane that covers the eyeball.

Remedy #1
- 10 chamomile buds, or 1 chamomile tea bag
- $\frac{1}{4}$ teaspoon salt
- 1 teaspoon eyebright (if available)

Gently clean the eye with a tissue that has been dipped in water that was boiled and cooled to lukewarm. Prepare an eyewash by making a cup of chamomile tea: steep chamomile buds or chamomile tea bag in hot water for 15 minutes. Add salt to the tea, plus 1 teaspoon of eyebright, if available. When the solution has cooled to lukewarm, pour it into an eyecup or shot glass. Put your eye down over the glass, press the glass against your face, and lift your head. Keep the eye open while the solution bathes the eye. Do this several times a day.

Remedy #2
- Aloe vera extract

Place 2 drops of aloe vera extract in the eye by pulling down the lower lid and putting drops under the lid.

Remedy #3
- 8 ounces water
- 1 teaspoon salt
- 1 tablespoon liquid glycerin

This remedy is for nose drops to be used when eye problems are accompanied by sinus problems. Nose drops can help open mucous membranes of the upper respiratory tract. Boil water, then let it cool to lukewarm. Add salt and liquid glycerin to the water. Place 10 drops into each nostril with the head held back so the drops can move through the entire nasal passage. This procedure can be repeated several times a day.

Tissue Salts

First stage of inflammation:

The *beginning* of a cold or allergy when there is tendency to fever, a runny nose with clear mucus, and eyes are red with burning sensation and feel gritty:

- *Ferrum phos.* 6X

On the first day, take 1 dose every $\frac{1}{2}$ hour (except when sleeping) until any of the symptoms change. If symptoms improve, lessen the number of doses to every 2 hours, but not for more than one day. Then, lessen the number of doses to 3 times daily for three additional days. If symptoms change from the first to the second stage, then stop this remedy and start using the remedies listed below.

Second stage of inflammation:

After the cold or inflammation has begun to settle and a yellowish crust forms on the eyelids, accompanied by soreness and irritation:

- *Natrum phos.* 6X
- *Kali sulph.* 6X

On the first day that symptoms are present, take 1 dose of both remedies every $1/2$ hour (except when sleeping) until any of the symptoms change. If symptoms improve, decrease the frequency of doses to every 2 hours, but not for more than a day. Then, decrease the number of doses to 3 times daily for three additional days.

Homeopathy

- *Euphrasia* 6X (D6 in Europe)

This remedy can be purchased at most health food stores in tablet or pill form. Take 1 dose every $1/2$ hour up to 5 times or until there is any change in the original symptoms. When any improvement occurs, decrease the number of doses to 1 every 3 hours for up to 12 hours. Then stop the cycle and see if the improvement continues through the next 24 hours. You can repeat the cycle if symptoms recur.

RED SWELLING ON EYELID

Our eyelashes not only protect our eyes from foreign particles but, more importantly, function as sensitive receivers of information from subtle impulses in our environment. These impulses make the entire visual function of the eye more sensitive. Eyelashes, like all hair, grow from follicles. Sometimes these follicles become inflamed or get infected—this is called a sty. There is a red, painful swelling like a small pimple or boil, often with a head of white pus. As soon as this boil ripens and bursts, the pain will disappear. General swelling of the eyelids can also be treated by the procedures listed below.

General Remedies

Remedy #1

- $1/2$ cup of water
- 1 teaspoon salt

Boil water, then dissolve salt in the water. Let it cool to lukewarm. Soak a cotton ball in the lukewarm solution, close the eye, and gently swab the eyelid. Repeat every 30 minutes for 2 hours.

Remedy #2
- Castor oil

Put $\frac{1}{2}$ teaspoon of castor oil on a cotton ball and place it over the eye for 1 hour. You can repeat this every other hour up to 6 times.

Remedy #3
- 2 teaspoons chamomile tea
- 1 teaspoon eyebright
- $\frac{1}{4}$ teaspoon salt

Combine chamomile tea with eyebright. Add the salt. Soak a cotton ball in the tea, close the eye, and gently swab the eyelid. Repeat every 30 minutes 2 hours.

Tissue Salts
- *Silicea* 6X
- *Ferrum phos.* 6X

Take these remedies together 3–5 times daily for up to three days. Reduce the number of doses as symptoms begin to improve.

GENERAL CARE OF THE EYE

Spices, Herbs, and Foods

- **Asparagus**
  THERAPEUTIC ACTION: Helps blurred, hazy, or weak vision; alleviates dryness and pain in the eyes; relieves irritated eyelids
  PREPARATION METHOD: Include in the daily diet
- **Black pepper**
  THERAPEUTIC ACTION: Strengthens vision
  PREPARATION METHOD: Include in the daily diet
- **Chicory**
  THERAPEUTIC ACTION: Reduces floaters
  PREPARATION METHOD: Standard hot infusion, decoction
- **Fennel seed**
  THERAPEUTIC ACTION: Reduces inflammation and conjunctivitis; strengthens eyesight; clears eyes
  PREPARATION METHOD: Standard hot infusion, decoction; can use tea as an eyewash

Reflexology

For instructions on reflexology, see "Reflexology" under "How to Use the Therapy Section" at the beginning of Part II.

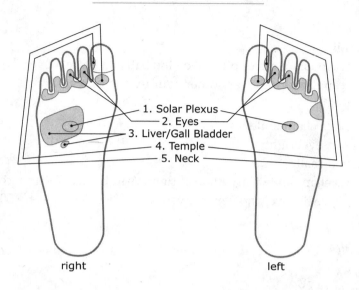

1. Solar Plexus
2. Eyes
3. Liver/Gall Bladder
4. Temple
5. Neck

right   left

FEVER

TEACHING

Fever is a natural response of the immune system and is the first and most important stage of the body healing itself. Fever can be external (affecting the whole body), internal (affecting organ and tissue systems), or local (affecting a specific area).

Fever occurs as a healing response to any stressor that compromises the body's functions and integrity. A stressor by definition is *any* factor that impacts the body or mind and that the organism cannot integrate. The immune system is in reality an integration system that mobilizes the healing mechanisms of the body and mind, making it possible to process what is occurring in the organism. Fever is one of the first responses initiated by the immune system to facilitate this healing and integration process.

None of us is able to integrate all of the events and factors to which we are exposed. For example, exposure to more extreme climatic conditions, such as too much heat, dampness, cold, or wind, often creates immune responses as the body attempts to deal with these situations. Other factors that can become stressors are the presence of toxins from old unresolved disease processes; recurring infections after use of antibiotics; side effects from drugs, vaccines, and dental amalgam toxins; environmental and food toxins; and traumatic emotional events.

Basically, fevers help the body accomplish a number of things. First, a fever increases biological heat. All processes in living organisms are supported by heat. Factors that we can't integrate produce cold responses that affect these biological processes, but fever counteracts these cold responses. We can see this pattern more clearly when we consider what happens during a shock response to an event. When something affects us very strongly and we can't immediately integrate it, we may become pale and cold. As we recover, we regain our warmth and color. Biological heat sustains the life and well-being of the organism as a whole; fever immediately counters cold processes by creating greater heat.

Secondly, fever increases the functions and reactions of the mucous membranes, and in so doing creates a higher metabolic, transforming activity in the tissues. The mucous membranes are the first tissues to react to factors that compromise the body. By increasing their activity, fever contributes to the body's healing processes.

All influences that compromise the body affect cells and tissues and can damage them or inhibit their biological functions. By increasing biological heat and stimulating the mucous membranes, fever helps activate and increase biological fluids. Just as heat is imperative for the functions of living organisms, so fluids are necessary for the life of cells and tissues. These fluids contain nutrients that build cells and immune substances that help protect and repair cells.

As fever stimulates biological heat and fluids, it also contributes through these same mechanisms to the elimination of toxins from the body. Fever activates *all* functions of the immune system, which is responsible for the stabilizing and integrating processes of the body and mind. One of these processes is cleansing the body of toxins that compromise the cells and tissues. We can see this in a simple example with which we are all familiar. When a fever breaks, we usually sweat quite profusely. Sweating is a response to the fever when it has reached the point of resolution and now needs to cleanse the tissues of the waste products formed during the healing processes. These wastes include dead cells and microbes, used fluids, and spent immune substances.

During fever, we notice other cleansing reactions. We tend to cough, which shows the body is eliminating wastes through the lungs. We know that we must drink considerable water during fever, not to counteract the fever but to help it eliminate toxins.

Microbes and the Immune Process

Microbes play an important role in the immune system's integrating and healing responses. Fascinating forms of life, microbes are fully individual living organisms with their own DNA and complex cell processes. They are the oldest life forms and the foundation and basis of all life on this planet. In addition, they are directly involved in *all* of nature's processes, from creating the living qualities of the soil, which supports all life, to assisting and governing the way cells and tissue systems function in animals and humans.

Initially, microbes assist our healing mechanisms by stimulating the immune system to respond to any factor that seriously affects the healthy functioning of our cells and tissues. To understand this process, we need to see how microbes interact with our cells. Microbes come into contact with our cells through their cell membranes, their outer covering. The cell membranes of microbes contain what are called "antigens," biochemical components that create signals causing the immune system to respond by initiating the body's healing mechanisms, which include fever, cleansing, and repair.

It is important to note that microbes appear as a *response* to factors that compromise or damage tissues and cells. They are not the original *cause* of the disease, but rather stimulate and activate our immune responses. We can see how microbes enter into the healing process through the simple example of strep throat, which involves the *Streptococcus* bacteria. In the first phase of what will become strep throat, the body's cell and tissue functions are affected by factors that they cannot integrate. As a result, mucous membranes are burdened beyond what they can deal with. They undergo subtle bioenergetic changes in their functions that specifically correspond to the metabolic energy fields of the *Streptococcus* bacteria, which is normally in contact with our systems. This change of energy fields alters the relationship between our cells and the bacteria. Our cells react to the antigens in the cell membrane of the bacteria, initiating immune responses that include fever and heightened mucous membrane activity.

The first phase of all acute disorders involves only symptoms that reflect the initial impacts of the stressors. These symptoms may include tiredness, restlessness, lack of appetite, and low spirits. It is in the second phase of acute disorders that the familiar symptoms of fever, phlegm, swelling of mucous membranes, and pain occurs. If you took a blood test in the first phase of the disorder, no bacteria would be present. Yet if you took a blood test during the second phase, bacteria would be present. Conversely, if the body is able to resolve the impact of the stressors during the first phase, the bacteria will never activate and the symptoms will resolve and proceed no further.

Fevers and Cold

Fever, then, is a natural part of what we experience when we have an acute condition like a cold. The term *cold* refers to the body's response to being chilled after exposure to cold weather, winds, or drafts. Cold air and drafts, or the Cold Phase of emotional stress, produce drying effects on cells, which compromise their natural fluid nature; cold temperatures or stress can lower the vital biological warmth of the cells. A decrease in fluids and biological heat disperses and fragments the cell's functional energies.

We must remember that all biological processes are by nature warm and moist. When conditions occur that are the opposite of the natural warmth and fluid processes, they inhibit our health. If this happens, the immune system will become active and produce conditions that help re-balance the system. We can see this reaction in the heat produced by fever and the phlegm produced in the mucous membranes that counteract the drying and cold factors.

An outdated concept in conventional medical practice maintains that fevers are "diseases," and need to be suppressed or treated. Consequently, fever suppressants like aspirin or other drugs are often used at the onset of fever. It is very important, however, *not* to suppress fevers because they are a foundation of the body's healing system. When we suppress fevers, we counteract the body's own healing mechanisms and the work of the immune system. It is better to use natural therapies that support the immune system, rather than therapies that suppress the fever.

THERAPY

When fevers are high and last for several days, we can assist the healing process by relieving the surface symptoms of fever by following the suggestions below. This is not the same thing as suppressing the fever mechanism itself; it simply provides greater comfort and helps the body resolve its issues more quickly.

Fevers strongly stimulate all bodily processes and healing mechanisms, including the senses. Therefore, it's a good idea to reduce all other forms of stimulation that could affect the body, such as strong light, loud noises, and movement. People with fever need loving care and attention given with encouragement and confidence. They don't need television, computer games, loud music, or excessive worry about being sick. The body needs rest and quiet to accomplish its healing. Do not wake a person to give them remedies; sleep enhances the healing process. For children especially, the emotional atmosphere should be calm and supportive, rather than fearful and overly concerned. A peaceful, loving, and confident presence contributes strongly to the healing process. If the child can tolerate quiet diversions, an adult might tell a good story or read a soothing book to the child.

Adults and children with a fever need to avoid eating heavy foods. Also, the body cannot digest large amounts of food when concentrating its activities on healing and restoring balance. Drinking plenty of water aids the cleansing process. In cases of high fever, drink only fluids and avoid eating because the body partially closes down digestive processes during fevers in order to use the energy usually used on digestion to enhance the healing processes. With milder fevers, or when the body begins to regain some of its natural appetite, herbal teas, broths, and unbuttered toast can be eaten as well.

After the fever has subsided and the body is returning to its normal functions, a feeling of well-being and an increased appetite will usually follow. It's best not to rush into heavy meals in this first improvement phase but to continue to eat sparingly—you can add normal food items, but add them in smaller quantities until the symptoms are completely resolved.

Remember that children normally produce higher fever than adults. This is natural because a child's developing body has a higher tissue metabolism than that of an adult in order to promote their growth and development.

The treatment suggestions for fever listed below support the immune system via the body's healing mechanisms and naturally reduce fever and its duration by speeding up the healing process.

General Remedies

Remedy #1
• For children and adults (not infants), place a cold towel under the back of the neck and under the calves of the legs. Remove when no longer cool. For very high fever, repeat every 20 minutes. For medium fever, repeat every hour.

Remedy #2
• Soak cotton socks or a towel in apple cider vinegar and place around the feet and up over the ankles. Leave in place for 2 hours and repeat until fever begins to decrease. Apple cider vinegar draws fever from the head, soothes the nerves, and increases circulation.

Remedy #3
• For children and adults (not infants), wrap an ice cube in a single layer of cloth and apply to the underside of the big toe for 30 seconds. Repeat every 20–30 minutes.

Remedy #4
• Sponge bathe the patient with room temperature water, letting the water

evaporate by uncovering the body until dry. Cover the body again after the water dries to prevent chills. The evaporation process will cool the body.

Remedy #5

• Shred large pieces of lettuce into a cup. Pour boiling water into the cup and let it steep for 15 minutes. Strain and sweeten the liquid with a little honey. Drink 2–4 cups daily.

Tissue Salts

For all fevers, use:

• *Ferrum phos.* 6X

If fever rises at night, add:

• *Kali sulph.* 6X

If fever is high and accompanied by weakness and exhaustion, add:

• *Kali phos.* 6X
• *Calc. phos.* 6X

Take these remedies every 30 minutes up to 8 times on the first day. For the next two days, take appropriate remedies 4–6 times per day. Reduce the number of doses as symptoms begin to improve.

Spices, Herbs, and Foods

The following are anti-inflammatory and help reduce fever at all stages.

• **Apple**
  PREPARATION METHOD: Fruit juice; include grated apple in the diet
• **Basil**
  PREPARATION METHOD: Standard hot infusion
• **Garlic**
  PREPARATION METHOD: Compress, herbal oil, garlic oil (apply these on symptomatic areas of the body, such as the chest, during a cold)
• **Ginger**
  PREPARATION METHOD: Standard hot infusion, decoction, fresh plant tincture, dry plant tincture
• **Onion**
  PREPARATION METHOD: Compress (apply to symptomatic area; check every 15 minutes and remove if the skin becomes red)
• **Pineapple**
  PREPARATION METHOD: Fruit juice
• **Sage**
  PREPARATION METHOD: Standard hot infusion, decoction, fresh plant tincture, dry plant tincture

Reflexology

For instructions on reflexology, see "Reflexology" under "How to Use the Therapy Section" at the beginning of Part II.

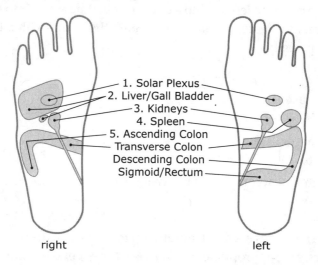

1. Solar Plexus
2. Liver/Gall Bladder
3. Kidneys
4. Spleen
5. Ascending Colon
Transverse Colon
Descending Colon
Sigmoid/Rectum

right   left

HEADACHE

TEACHING

You're probably beginning to understand that Classical medicine views the functions of the body quite differently from conventional medicine. A classically trained doctor usually will attribute the cause of symptoms that manifest in one area of the body to disturbances—or imbalances—located in a different part of the body. The same theoretical approach applies to headaches.

Three organ systems may play a part in headaches: the Liver/Gallbladder System, the Kidney/Bladder System, and the Stomach/Spleen System. All three systems control the tissues of the scalp, the skull, and the brain. As with all the organ systems of the body, they are composed of a network of energy channels, called *meridians* in Traditional Chinese Medicine and *nadis* in Ayurvedic medicine. The meridians of the Gallbladder System and the Bladder System cover the entire head and extend into the cerebral cortex, the small brain (cerebellum), and the brain stem (medulla oblongata), as well as the eyes. The Stomach System controls the lower sinuses, the teeth roots, the jaw, and some of the eye functions.

If there are chronic functional health issues in any of these three systems, it will cause disturbances in the circulation of the blood in the inner tissues of the head, impinge on local nerves, and create high energy levels in the tissues that result in pain. Simple headaches and migraines are caused by a number of different factors connected with the functions of these organ systems. Chronic issues such as eyestrain, digestive problems, urinary and reproductive system issues, problems with the teeth, muscle tension, poor vertebral alignment, and problems with the sinuses can all create headaches. Toxins from mercury fillings in the teeth as well as root canals, poorly fitting bridgework, or a misaligned bite are often overlooked as causes of headaches.

In cases of chronic headache or migraine, it is important to contact your natural healthcare professional to find a natural solution to the *cause* of the problem. Taking painkilling medications is *not* a real solution to the problem because this approach will compromise the body, due to the side effects of these medications. Traumas such as concussion or whiplash will also produce headaches and can have other serious consequences. If you have had a concussion or blow to the head, consult your doctor as soon as possible to determine if emergency care is required.

THERAPY

SINUS HEADACHE

Herbs and Spices
- Ginger powder

Mix 2 tablespoons of warm water with enough ginger powder to make a paste. Apply to the forehead for 30 minutes. The warming sensation will not be harmful.

HEADACHES IN THE TEMPLES

General Remedies
Remedy #1
- Chamomile tea
- $\frac{1}{4}$ teaspoon cumin (if available)
- $\frac{1}{4}$ teaspoon coriander (if available)

Prepare a cup of chamomile tea. Add the cumin and coriander, if you have them. Drink 1 cup 3 times per day.

Remedy #2
- Castor oil (fresh)

Rub castor oil into your temples.

HEADACHE IN THE BACK OF THE HEAD

General Remedies

Remedy #1
- Juice of $\frac{1}{2}$ a lemon
- 8 ounces water
- 1 teaspoon olive oil
- 1 pinch of of ginger powder

Squeeze lemon juice into water. Add olive oil and ginger powder. Drink once daily.

Remedy #2
- Olive oil
- Ginger powder

Make a paste of ginger powder and olive oil and apply it to the large bone behind the ears. Leave in place for 30 minutes. Apply 3 times daily.

HEADACHE IN FRONT OF THE HEAD

General Remedies

Remedy #1
- Chili or cayenne pepper
- Olive oil

Crush chilies (or use powdered cayenne). Mix with enough olive oil to form a paste. Apply to the site (avoid getting near the eyes).

GASTRIC HEADACHES AND HEADACHES FROM GASTRIC TOXINS

General Remedies

Remedy #1
- $\frac{1}{4}$ teaspoon cumin
- $\frac{1}{4}$ teaspoon coriander
- 8 ounces boiling water

Mix cumin and coriander. Pour boiling water over the mixture. Let steep for 5 minutes. Drink 1 glass 3 times per day.

> **Technique for Increasing Circulation:** There will usually be more air coming in through one nostril than the other. With the thumb and forefinger, close off the nostril that has more air coming through it and breathe through the other nostril until the headache is reduced.

Nervous Tension Headache

Tissue Salts

- *Kali phos.* 6X
- *Mag. phos.* 6X
- *Calc. phos.* 6X
- *Silicea* 6X

Take these remedies together 3 times daily for up to four days. Reduce the number of doses as symptoms improve.

Headaches with Gastric Upset

Tissue Salts

- *Kali mur.* 6X
- *Natrum sulph.* 6X
- *Natrum phos.* 6X
- *Calc. sulph.* 6X

Take these remedies together 3 times daily for up to four days. Reduce the number of doses as symptoms improve.

General Care of Headaches

Spices and Herbs

- **Bay Leaf**
  THERAPEUTIC ACTION: Relieves all headaches
  PREPARATION METHOD: Standard hot infusion, decoction, dry plant tincture
- **Chicory**
  THERAPEUTIC ACTION: Relieves gastric headaches and migraines
  PREPARATION METHOD: Standard hot infusion, decoction, fresh plant tincture, dry plant tincture
- **Ginger and turmeric** (use together)
  THERAPEUTIC ACTION: Relieves all headaches
  PREPARATION METHOD: Standard hot infusion, dry plant tincture
- **Marjoram**
  THERAPEUTIC ACTION: Relieves migraines
  PREPARATION METHOD: Standard hot infusion, decoction, fresh plant tincture, dry plant tincture
- **Rosemary**
  THERAPEUTIC ACTION: For all headaches; supports circulation

PREPARATION METHOD: Standard hot infusion, decoction, fresh plant tincture, dry plant tincture

Reflexology

For instructions on reflexology, see "Reflexology" under "How to Use the Therapy Section" at the beginning of Part II.

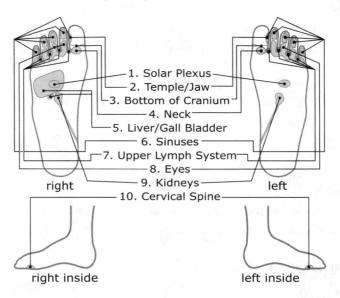

1. Solar Plexus
2. Temple/Jaw
3. Bottom of Cranium
4. Neck
5. Liver/Gall Bladder
6. Sinuses
7. Upper Lymph System
8. Eyes
9. Kidneys
10. Cervical Spine

right   left

right inside   left inside

HEART AILMENTS

TEACHING

The development of the heart in the embryo is quite a remarkable story because it reveals how the heart functions as an integral part of the body and mind. The heart develops from the first blood cells and blood vessels in the fetus. These blood cells develop from the embryonic tissue system called the mesoderm. This tissue system controls the *balance* between the functions of the digestive tract, which nourishes the body's cells, and the nerve system, which is a communication network that carries the signals from our mental, emotional, and physical processes to all the systems of the body. The blood vessels, on the other hand, develop from the embryonic tissue system called the endoderm, which produces our glands and intestinal tract. The fact that the heart develops originally from the blood cells is important in that it is the blood that pumps the heart, not the heart that pumps the blood. (This is why a person can die if they bleed too heavily, even though the nerve system that is connected to the heart is not damaged.)

To help understand this concept, look at the red blood cells. They contain two important elements, copper and iron, which help cells take up oxygen from foods and the air we breathe. Copper has a rhythmical energy that expands and contracts in all physiological processes, very much like the beat of the heart. Oxygen, in turn, contains a strong bioenergetic component that stimulates all biological processes and enhances the rhythmical work of copper. When breathing problems deplete the body's level of oxygen, the body either functions poorly and has little energy or can die from oxygen deprivation. Sometimes simple breathing exercises produce an almost immediate sense of new energy and revitalize the body.

The heart's pumping action is caused by the contraction and relaxation in its muscle system. The muscles contract or relax depending on the signals from the nerves connected to the muscle tissue. Nerve tissues are basically electrical in that their signals are bioelectrical charges that are stimulated by the bioenergetic component found in the oxygen molecules of the blood. The electrical charges flow along the nerve threads like current in a wire, stimulating the nerve centers in the heart and causing the muscles to contract and pump the blood.

It is important to note that the heart and lungs work together in a partnership. The heart sends blood directly to the lungs to be recharged with the primary biological energy of oxygen. This primary bioenergy controls all aspects of life through its rhythm of contracting and expanding, taking hold of processes and letting them go, a rhythm that is reflected in our breathing. Notice that all biological processes have cyclical rhythms, such as activity and sleep, inhaling and exhaling, the rhythm of the heartbeat, eating and eliminating, and muscles tensing in work and then relaxing. Throughout days, nights, and seasons, rhythms dominate all of nature. Without this taking in and letting go, receiving and giving, we could not function.

The Heart Center

The heart muscle is the only organ of the body that has two kinds of basic muscle tissue—muscle tissue like those we use to move our bodies and muscle tissue similar to those found in our inner organs. This means that the heart, which contains both kinds of muscles, is involved directly with the inner processes of life that move from system to system, as well as the outer movements of our life as we experience the world.

All cultures consider the heart to be the center of the individual. We associate love and all our emotions with the heart. When we have strong emotions, we notice an immediate change in our pulse. For centuries, the criterion for death was a stopped heartbeat (even though the nerve system, for instance, was still alive). We speak of "a change of heart" when the spiritual aspect of our being is discovering new ways of responding to situations that profoundly affect our lives. In the Christian tradition, the word *conversion* is translated from the Greek word *metanoia* meaning "change of heart." All Classical medical traditions identify the heart as the center of human consciousness and spirituality. The heart represents the true self and the foundation of the mind.

Heart Health Issues

According to Classical medicine, most heart problems are not *caused* by the heart; the symptoms merely appear in the heart. The main causes of most heart problems originate in the Liver/Gallbladder System. Heart problems stem mainly from issues involving circulation, like clogging of the arteries, failure of veins, nerve center problems, or problems caused by blocked energies, especially in the Gallbladder System, which Classical medicine identifies as having a special relationship to the function of the heart.

The production of plaque that clogs arteries can be attributed mainly to digestive problems in the Liver System, where food is not completely digested and forms a heavy, gluey material that circulates in the blood. This material is composed mostly of calcium, cholesterol, and fibrin, a substance that helps clot blood when we cut ourselves. The liver also strongly influences the circulation of blood through the veins.

Energetically, the heart is strongly influenced by the Gallbladder System, which affects the muscle tissues of the heart. Together with the liver, the gallbladder controls a number of functions in the body related to the heart, including those of the reproductive organs, as well as the heart's protective sheath, called the pericardium, which influences certain aspects of the sexual hormones (in the Chinese medical tradition, the uterus is called "the little heart"). The brain stem and spinal nerves contain nerve centers that connect to the heart and the Liver/Gallbladder System also energetically controls these nerve systems.

Often, symptoms like heart palpitations, a feeling of pressure on the heart, and pain around the heart are caused by digestive disturbances. The heart lies very close to the top of the diaphragm. The stomach, liver, and intestines that lie underneath can press up against the diaphragm. During the digestive process, gas may form and put pressure on the diaphragm muscle that then presses up against the nerves that enervate both the heart and the digestive organs. This pressure can cause heart symptoms. The diaphragm has a small opening in it that allows the nerves, blood vessels, and esophagus to pass through to the organs below. Many people have a small hernia or tear in this opening of the diaphragm muscle, a condition called a hiatal hernia, that tends to increase heart symptoms. Heart symptoms should be diagnosed by a doctor to ensure that there is nothing wrong with the heart organ itself that requires special attention.

Conventional medicine often uses the measurement of blood pressure to evaluate the heart's function. This procedure measures the relative pressure of the blood flowing between the artery system and the vein system of the body. The doctor will tell you, for example, that you have a blood pressure that measures 150 over 100 (written 150/100). The first number, called the *systolic pressure,* refers to the pressure relative to the artery system that conducts blood outward from the heart to the rest of the body. The second number, called the *diastolic pressure,* refers to the relative pressure of blood circulation in the veins that return the blood from the organs and tissues to the heart.

Many people today take medicines for high blood pressure. Though these medicines are usually successful in reducing blood pressure, they do not deal with the *cause* of high blood pressure and they often create side effects. As stated above, the causes of high blood pressure usually are not caused by the heart itself. According to Classical medicine, high blood pressure can be caused by chronic gastric ailments (which can also cause plaque buildup), by anything that affects the reproductive organs, and by misalignment of the neck vertebrae, which impedes the nerve system. Misalignment can affect the small brain and spinal cord that have centers controlling the nerve functions of the heart and the circulation. If you have high blood pressure, it is a good idea to consult your natural healthcare professional and have the problem assessed.

One of the problems concerning high blood pressure medicine is the way it is prescribed. A patient's blood pressure is taken routinely during a visit to the doctor's office. If the blood pressure readings are high, the doctor is likely to prescribe drugs to lower the blood pressure. Blood pressure, like all other functions of the body, varies during the day depending on the conditions of the organ systems and your activities. You might just be peaking at the time the pressure is tested. If it was taken some hours later, it would be lower. Also, it has been confirmed that most people's blood pressure increases to a certain extent when in the doctor's office. The surest way to determine if blood pressure medicine is necessary is to purchase a good quality blood-pressure-measuring device and take your blood pressure morning, noon, and evening for one month. Write down your readings. If, as an adult, your blood pressure remains high, meaning the top number is *consistently* higher than 150 and the lower number is *consistently* higher than 95, then you should consider seeing your natural healthcare provider or a medical doctor.

THERAPY

General Remedies

Remedy to Enhance Circulation:

- Garlic

Consume garlic in the daily diet—raw, baked, or fried. You can also prepare a fresh plant tincture.

Remedy to Reduce Plaque:

- 3 lemons
- 30 peeled garlic cloves
- 1 quart of distilled water

Scrape off and discard the outer yellow layer of the peel from the lemons; allow the white rind underneath to remain. Slice the lemons. Place lemon slices in a blender with the peeled garlic cloves and blend. Add the mixture to the distilled water and bring slowly to a boil and simmer for five minutes. Let the mixture cool and then strain. Pour the strained juice into a clean bottle and refrigerate. Drink 1 ounce 2 hours before or after your evening meal for three weeks. Pause for eight days, then repeat for three more weeks. Do this once yearly. **Note: This is not for children. Also, do not take flu vaccine while on this regimen.**

Remedy to Lower Cholesterol and Reduce Plaque:

- Fresh ginger

Prepare a standard hot infusion, fresh plant tincture, or herbal wine. In addition, consume ginger in the daily diet.

Remedy to Enhance Circulation and Reduce Plaque:

- Pineapple juice or fresh pineapple

Consume pineapple juice or fresh pineapple daily.

Reflexology

For instructions on reflexology, see "Reflexology" under "How to Use the Therapy Section" at the beginning of Part II.

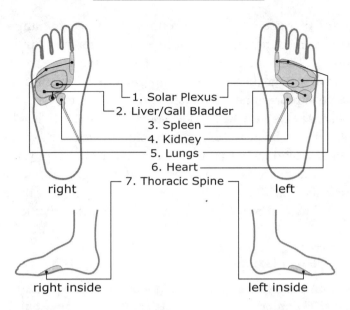

right   1. Solar Plexus   left

2. Liver/Gall Bladder
3. Spleen
4. Kidney
5. Lungs
6. Heart
7. Thoracic Spine

right inside   left inside

INFANT CARE

TEACHING

Life is a process of evolution during which the body and mind continually grow and mature. The transformative aspects of growth occur due to a continual relationship between the individual and the environment. We usually think of the environment as that which surrounds us and which our senses perceive. The environment of life, however, is this and much more. It includes the factors of our emotional spaces, nature with its climate and landscapes, and the entire cosmos with its highly dynamic energies that have created the planets and stars. In order to live and thrive in this environment brimming with transformation, growth, and development, a child must be allowed to create programs in the body and mind that accommodate life experiences.

When a newborn's umbilical cord is cut, that child becomes a fully independent person and embarks on a uniquely personal life journey. During the first stage of this journey, which is childhood, the care and attention that a child receives will serve as a foundation for his or her entire life. Love, care, and attention are the foundations of life because all of life's actions and responses are based on the essential human quality of being able to care.

Through the first year, the infant acquires his or her first impressions of life, which are formed through relationships to the people and the features of his environment. These impressions help inherent aspects of the child's identity to form and become manifest. It is important that these first impressions convey a sense of peacefulness, love, attention, and caring.

A child's senses are very acute. The sounds and activity levels that surround a baby should be peaceful and harmonious. He or she should receive quality, focused attention. In traditional cultures, creating a physical sense of well-being for the infant is done through a daily light oil massage of the whole body. This type of touch stimulates the development of the nerve system and other physical organs as well as provides a sense of love, contact, and care.

Childhood Health Issues

During the first ten years of life, a child's body is growing and developing new skills. The mind is expanding its abilities to manage and focus experiences and learning how to respond to its own needs as well as to the needs of others. In this developmental stage, the immune system builds its capacity to integrate internal and external influences that affect the body, mind, and spirit. The relationships inherent in the child's physical and emotional environment stimulate and train the immune system and its responses in cleansing the body, supporting tissue functions, and integrating emotional responses.

The immune system reveals its ongoing work of integration and support primarily through activity in the mucous membranes, which are most active during this period of childhood. This heightened activity occurs because the mucous membranes are connected by functional energies to the digestive system and the lymph system. These systems are both connected to the processes concerned with the building-up and maintenance of the body's cells and tissues.

During the first five years of childhood, parents often become concerned when their child suddenly develops a fever or symptoms such as sore throat, ear infection, or bronchitis. With few exceptions, these symptoms reflect activities of the immune system as it cleanses and strengthens the body. As we have indicated, the immune system is really an *integration* system—immune activities serve to help infants in continually integrating all of the new experiences to which they are exposed.

Most toxins found in infants stem from processes that occur during the fetal stage, prior to birth. The fetal child becomes burdened with the same toxins that burden the mother—toxins found in substances such as nonorganic foods, chlorinated water, medicines, cosmetics, household cleaners, and dental amalgams. The bacteria from root canals can also produce toxins that travel from the mother's tissues into the fetal child's systems.

We must remember that the child's own physiological life begins only after the umbilical cord is cut and he inhales his first independent breath. After birth, the infant must begin his own life with all of its physical, mental, and emotional processes. Childhood is both a period of activation of these processes and the period in which they develop. New emotional and social experiences also need to be integrated into the child's growing world. The immune system is responsible for integrating these experiences. A certain amount of stress inevitably accompanies a child's development, and the immune system is primarily involved in the integration processes that resolve stress. As mentioned above, initial immune responses are visible through the activity of the mucous membranes, but deeper processes involving the digestive system, which build and nourish both the body and mind, are active as well.

Symptoms like fever and the production of mucus are signs that the immune system is at work and "programming" the body for how to best respond to its new environment. The symptoms, therefore, are not diseases but part of the process of development and growth. They should not be treated by drugs that will suppress these immune activities, but rather through natural means that will support the child's integration processes and development.

In the same sense, childhood diseases such as chicken pox, mumps, and measles are not really "diseases" in the normal sense of the word but contribute to the health of the body. We call them "childhood diseases" because they normally occur during the first ten years of life. Since childhood diseases play a vital role in the development of the organism as a whole, we might call them "nature's vaccines." These "diseases" contribute to the child's health in two important ways. First, they stimulate immunity and provide new codes and response patterns that the immune system will use to deal with possible future diseases. In addition, all disease patterns contain emotional dimensions along with their physical aspects. Therefore, childhood diseases also help the immune system create new integration responses for the child's emerging intellect and emotional responses. We need to better understand the role that childhood diseases play in our health and development and not suppress them with vaccines.

In the United States, childhood diseases are still considered pathological and something to fear and conquer. Conventional medicine has a vast vaccination program to eradicate and prevent their occurrence. This approach, of course, defeats nature's purpose in using the "disease" process to help the organism grow and develop. In European countries, many parents opt not to have their children vaccinated. They actually set up contagion groups in which children can be exposed to peers who have a disease. These parents recognize the value of childhood diseases in the ongoing health of their children.

Vaccines

Fear and ignorance play a major role in the vaccine issue. Many parents say that when they spoke with their doctor about forgoing their child's vaccines, the doctor's response was akin to "Do you know what you're doing? Do you want to be responsible for your child dying from one of these diseases?" After such a reply, only the most informed parents will choose not to vaccinate.

Virtually all deaths from childhood diseases occur *only* when the child's immune system is so severely compromised by previous factors that it cannot integrate or support the immune processes that accompany the disease. The factors that compromise and weaken the immune system include abuse, lack of proper care and nourishment, toxic burdens from previous vaccines, chemical drugs, poor food, chronic allergies, and unresolved health issues.

Two main problems with vaccines warrant consideration. First, though vaccines produce antibodies, they do not create immunity through the cellular immune system. Cellular immune mechanisms are much more important than antibodies when dealing with disease. Antibodies work on the biochemical levels of microbes and help neutralize microbes but do not affect the immune functions of the body's cells. As we have discussed, microbes do not *cause* disease but rather are a part of the resolution processes going on in our immune system. True health lies not in being able to fight off microbes but in the stability of our cell and tissue functions. This can be seen by the fact that many people who are vaccinated get the disease at some point even *after* being vaccinated.

The second factor pertains to the way vaccines are delivered to the body. Our immune systems are designed to interface between the outside influences of the environment and the inside functions of the body. The tissues that create this interface are the mucous membranes and the skin. Only these tissues are in direct contact with the outer world. The concept of contagion in conventional medicine states that we become sick when we come into contact with a pathogenic microbe. This contact has to occur initially through the skin or the mucous membranes of the lungs or digestive tract. Most vaccines are injected directly into the body, bypassing the essential immune mechanisms located in the skin and mucous membranes. This means that the immune system has no programmed way of integrating the foreign substances in the vaccine, which include pathological microbes, preservatives, and foreign proteins that are all toxic and put a great burden on the body. Many homeopaths and naturopaths have noticed in their practice that children suffering from diverse immune problems such as eczema, asthma, attention deficit problems, and hyperactivity have been helped when the burdens of previous vaccines are resolved through natural therapies.

To put it simply, we can say that a vaccine reproduces the *dynamic pattern* of a disease in the body but without creating the disease itself. This pattern creates chronic functional disturbances deep in the body's systems that in time create other symptoms. For example, a hepatitis vaccine will create the underlying subtle patterns of hepatitis in the body but there will be no hepatitis virus present if a blood test were taken. Because hepatitis is a liver disease, the liver system will be compromised and its energy functions chronically disturbed, creating symptoms throughout its system that can emerge anywhere, from skin problems to symptoms that disturb central nervous system functions and hormone balance. Though no hepatitis virus is present, a pulse diagnosis such as used in Chinese medicine or an iris diagnosis as used in naturopathic practice would show definite signs of a chronically compromised liver system.

Somehow in all of this, conventional medicine has never observed the fact that, statistically, more children suffer from health issues like autism, attention deficit disorder, and autoimmune disorders than they did fifty years ago. Although there have always been "allergies," asthma, eczema, and behavioral problems, the sheer number of children today who suffer from these ailments is at an extreme. This trend of increasing health issues follows the rising curve of the number and types of vaccines to which children are subjected. Sooner or later, we will make that connection.

Growth and Development

Nature provides the mechanisms of growth and development for the infant. These mechanisms have their own rate of change, and the healthiest way to provide care during growth is to allow the unfolding of the child's abilities in accordance with the natural rate of development and integration. In our culture, we often stimulate development in an inappropriate manner by pushing the child forward to develop more quickly than his body and mind can integrate. The drive for the child to excel in sports and learning on more advanced levels often compromises the child's natural development processes and serves only to satisfy adult ambitions. Unstructured play, free from competition, is an essential component in a child's growth, allowing the mind and emotions to develop in accordance with the child's unique needs and emerging personality. Overstructuring childhood development patterns inhibits the unfolding of the personality, including social skills and creativity, and can create chronic stress that will affect all later areas of development.

THERAPY

MEASLES

General Remedies

Remedy #1

- $\frac{1}{2}$ cup lentils (any variety)
- 1 teaspoon salt
- 1 teaspoon turmeric
- 1 quart of water

Make a broth by simmering the lentils, salt, and turmeric in water for 3 hours. Drink $\frac{1}{2}$ to 1 cup 2–3 times daily. This will soothe the throat and help bring out the rash.

Tissue Salts

- *Ferrum phos.* 6X
- *Kali mur.* 6X
- *Kali sulph.* 6X
- *Silicea* 6X

Give these remedies together 4–5 times daily for up to 3–4 days; reduce the number of doses as symptoms begin to improve.

Spices and Herbs

- **Ginger and turmeric** (mix together)

  THERAPEUTIC ACTION: Relieves headaches; strengthens the immune system; cleanses toxins

  PREPARATION METHOD: Standard hot infusion, dry plant tincture

- **Marjoram**

  THERAPEUTIC ACTION: Relieves headaches that often occur at the onset of measles

  PREPARATION METHOD: Standard hot infusion, decoction, fresh plant tincture, dry plant tincture

---

MUMPS

Tissue Salts

- *Ferrum phos.* 6X
- *Kali mur.* 6X
- *Natrum mur.* 6X

  Give these remedies together 4–5 times daily for up to 3–4 days; reduce the number of doses as symptoms begin to improve.

Spices and Herbs

- **Ginger and turmeric** (mix together)

  THERAPEUTIC ACTION: Relieves headache; strengthens the immune system; cleanses toxins

  PREPARATION METHOD: Standard hot infusion, dry plant tincture

---

SCARLET FEVER

Tissue Salts

For Rash:

- *Natrum sulph.* 6X
- *Kali sulph.* 6X
- *Kali mur.* 6X
- *Ferrum phos.* 6X

  Give these remedies together 4–5 times daily for up to 3–4 days; reduce the number of doses as symptoms begin to improve.

With Swollen Glands:

- *Silicea* 6X (add to above tissue salts)

Spices

- **Ginger and Turmeric** (mix together)

  THERAPEUTIC ACTION: Relieves headache; strengthens the immune system; cleanses toxins

  PREPARATION METHOD: Standard hot infusion, dry plant tincture

CHICKEN POX

Tissue Salts

First Stage Rash:
- *Ferrum phos.* 6X

Give these remedies together 4–5 times daily for up to 3–4 days; reduce the number of doses as symptoms begin to improve or change.

For Eruptions:
- *Kali mur.* 6X
- *Calc. sulph.* 6X
- *Natrum sulph.* 6X
- *Silicea* 6X

Give these remedies together 4–5 times daily for up to 3–4 days; reduce the number of doses as symptoms begin to improve.

Spices

- **Ginger and turmeric** (mix together)

THERAPEUTIC ACTION: Relieves headaches; strengthens the immune system; cleanses toxins

PREPARATION METHOD: Standard hot infusion, dry plant tincture

WHOOPING COUGH

Tissue Salts

- *Ferrum phos.* 6X
- *Kali mur.* 6X
- *Natrum mur.* 6X
- *Kali phos.* 6X
- *Kali sulph.* 6X
- *Mag. phos.* 6X
- *Calc. phos.* 6X

Give these remedies together 4–5 times daily for up to 3–4 days; reduce the number of doses as symptoms begin to improve.

Spices

- **Ginger and turmeric** (mix together)

THERAPEUTIC ACTION: Relieves headache; strengthens the immune system; cleanses toxins

PREPARATION METHOD: Standard hot infusion, dry plant tincture

To Calm and Relax Infants

General Remedies

Remedy #1
- Olive oil
Massage baby or child with olive oil at body temperature.

Tissue Salts

- *Calc. phos.* 6X
- *Mag. phos.* 6X
- *Kali phos.* 6X
Give these remedies together 1–2 times daily for up to four days.

Spices and Herbs

- **Anise seed**
THERAPEUTIC ACTION: Reduces colic and flatulence
PREPARATION METHOD: Standard hot infusion, decoction, fresh plant tincture
- **Caraway**
THERAPEUTIC ACTION: Reduces mucus in lungs and flatulence
PREPARATION METHOD: Standard hot infusion, decoction, fresh plant tincture
- **Chicory**
THERAPEUTIC ACTION: Reduces headache and digestive disturbances
PREPARATION METHOD: Standard hot infusion, decoction, fresh plant tincture, dry plant tincture
- **Fennel**
THERAPEUTIC ACTION: Sedative
PREPARATION METHOD: Standard hot infusion, decoction, fresh plant tincture
- **Rosemary**
THERAPEUTIC ACTION: Calming; strengthens the body's functions
PREPARATION METHOD: Standard hot infusion, decoction, fresh plant tincture, dry plant tincture

Bronchitis

General Remedies

For Infants:

Remedy #1
- $1/8$ teaspoon aloe vera gel
- Breast milk

Dissolve aloe vera gel in mother's breast milk. Give to infant three times per day while bronchial symptoms persist.

Remedy #2

- 1 teaspoon aloe vera gel
- $\frac{1}{2}$ cup warm water
Dissolve aloe gel in warm water and apply to chest.

For Toddlers:

- 1 clove of garlic, crushed
- 1 ounce olive oil
- 3 teaspoons honey
Prepare garlic oil by mixing a crushed garlic clove with olive oil. Let stand for 24 hours. Then mix 1 teaspoon of the garlic oil with the honey. Give the child $\frac{1}{2}$ teaspoon 3 times per day.

Tissue Salts

For First Stage of Bronchitis with Fever:

(continue using this tissue salt if fever continues into other stages):

- *Ferrum phos.* 6X
Give every hour up to 6 times per day for two days; reduce the number of doses as symptoms begin to improve.

For Second Stage of Bronchitis with White Phlegm:

- *Kali mur.* 6X
Give every hour up to 6 times a day for two days; reduce the number of doses as symptoms begin to improve.

For Third Stage of Bronchitis with Yellowish or Greenish Phlegm:

- *Calc. sulph.* 6X
- *Kali sulph.* 6X
- *Natrum sulph.* 6X
Give these remedies every hour up to 6 times a day for two days; reduce the number of doses as symptoms begin to improve.

Herbs

- **Caraway**
  THERAPEUTIC ACTION: Reduces mucus in lungs and reduces flatulence
  PREPARATION METHOD: Standard hot infusion, decoction, fresh plant tincture, dry plant tincture

- **Sage**
  THERAPEUTIC ACTION: Reduces fever
  PREPARATION METHOD: Herbal bath

Reflexology

For instructions on reflexology, see "Reflexology" under "How to Use the Therapy Section" at the beginning of Part II.

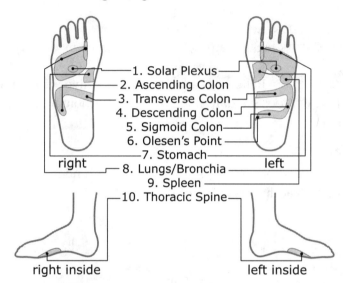

SIMPLE DIGESTIVE UPSETS

Tissue Salts

For colic:

- *Mag. phos.* 6X
- *Natrum phos.* 6X
- *Narum sulph.* 6X
- *Kali sulph.* 6X

Give these remedies together every 2 hours up to 5 times per day, reducing the number of doses as symptoms begin to improve. In chronic cases, these tissue salts can be given twice daily for 1–3 weeks.

For diarrhea:

- *Ferrum phos.* 6X
- *Natrum phos.* 6X
- *Calc. phos.* 6X
- *Silicea* 6X

Give these remedies together every 2 hours up to 5 times per day for up to two days, reducing the number of doses as symptoms begin to improve.

Spices and Herbs

- **Anise seed**
  THERAPEUTIC ACTION: Relieves colic and reduces flatulence
  PREPARATION METHOD: Standard hot infusion, decoction, fresh plant tincture
- **Bay leaf**
  THERAPEUTIC ACTION: Relieves headaches and digestive disturbances
  PREPARATION METHOD: Standard hot infusion, decoction, dry plant tincture
- **Chicory**
  THERAPEUTIC ACTION: Relieves headaches and digestive disturbances
  PREPARATION METHOD: Standard hot infusion, decoction, fresh plant tincture, dry plant tincture

Reflexology

For instructions on reflexology, see "Reflexology" under "How to Use the Therapy Section" at the beginning of Part II.

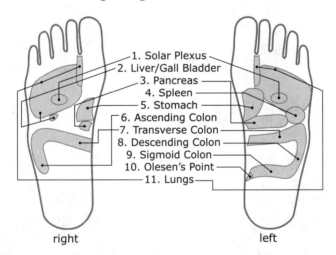

1. Solar Plexus
2. Liver/Gall Bladder
3. Pancreas
4. Spleen
5. Stomach
6. Ascending Colon
7. Transverse Colon
8. Descending Colon
9. Sigmoid Colon
10. Olesen's Point
11. Lungs

right   left

GENERAL INFANT CARE

Spices, Herbs, and Foods

- **Anise seed**
  THERAPEUTIC ACTION: Relieves colic and reduces flatulence
  PREPARATION METHOD: Standard hot infusion, decoction, fresh plant tincture

- **Bay leaf**

  THERAPEUTIC ACTION: Relieves headaches and digestive disturbances

  PREPARATION METHOD: Standard hot infusion, decoction, dry plant tincture

- **Caraway**

  THERAPEUTIC ACTION: Reduces mucus in lungs and flatulence

  PREPARATION METHOD: Standard hot infusion, decoction, fresh plant tincture

- **Carrots**

  THERAPEUTIC ACTION: Relieves diarrhea

  PREPARATION METHOD: Make a soup by peeling two large carrots and cutting into slices. Simmer in one quart of water in a covered pan for one hour. Give one ounce 2–4 times per day for an infant; give two ounces 2–4 times per day for toddlers.

- **Chicory**

  THERAPEUTIC ACTION: Relieves headaches and digestive disturbances

  PREPARATION METHOD: Standard hot infusion, decoction, fresh plant tincture, dry plant tincture

- **Fennel**

  THERAPEUTIC ACTION: Natural sedative and digestive aid

  PREPARATION METHOD: Standard hot infusion, decoction, fresh plant tincture

- **Ginger and turmeric**

  THERAPEUTIC ACTION: Relieves headaches; good combination remedy for all childhood diseases

  PREPARATION METHOD: Standard hot infusion, dry plant tincture

- **Marjoram**

  THERAPEUTIC ACTION: Relieves headaches; use at onset of measles

  PREPARATION METHOD: Standard hot infusion, decoction, fresh plant tincture, dry plant tincture

- **Rosemary**

  THERAPEUTIC ACTION: Calming; strengthens the body's functions

  PREPARATION METHOD: Standard hot infusion, decoction, fresh plant tincture, dry plant tincture

- **Sage**

  THERAPEUTIC ACTION: Reduces fever

  PREPARATION METHOD: Herbal bath

MUSCLE AND JOINT PAIN

TEACHING

In the classical traditions of medical science indigenous to China and India, the Liver/Gallbladder System is understood as controlling, among other processes, the function of the muscles, tendons, joints, and ligaments. The Liver/Gallbladder System relates to six major aspects of the body and mind: the Element of Space; the primary digestive metabolism and formation of bile; the control of the hormone system; the iron metabolism of the blood for the immune system and primary detoxification; the midbrain functions; and the ability to manifest oneself in an emotional and psychological sense. In Classical medicine, this last point is said to be the Liver/Gallbladder System's ability to "lay plans and strategies" that manifest the will of the individual.

These six areas that the Liver System controls may sound very different, but when we think carefully about them, we can see that the ability to make use of space—being able to move, create, and change things in the spaces around us like our homes, our communities, and our world—is directly connected to our ability to express and manifest who we truly are as individuals. It is our ability to transform, to metabolize energy from the food, air, and fluids of our environment, that enables us to live, and therefore creatively manifest who we are, building the visions and potentials of our lives.

A healthy liver function, then, has much to do with how our joints and muscles work. This in turn reflects our self-esteem and our ability to express who we really are. Anything that severely damages our self-esteem, for example, will affect the manifestation of who we truly are, and therefore decrease our desire and ability to move in our social environment. All of these factors affect the muscles and joints that we use to move through our world.

The Liver/Gallbladder System and the Muscles

The liver's functional partner is the gallbladder. The gallbladder is a very special organ in that it controls the large brain bark (cerebral cortex) and brain stem; important aspects of the heart; the hip joint; the secretion of bile; and, with the liver, functions of the reproductive organs, as well as muscles and joints. Psychologically, the gallbladder is associated with our will. The liver helps us plan and strategize, while the gallbladder enables us to put these plans into action.

When the Liver/Gallbladder System is compromised, the muscles become tense. If this tension is chronic, the muscles will create problems for the structural integrity of the body and its movements. Conversely, if the muscles and joints are compromised through work, exercise, or sports, the Liver/Gallbladder System will be functionally disturbed. The muscles that move our body work in pairs; your left arm has a bicep, for instance, as does your right arm. If you overuse the muscles on one side of the body, the other side will become weak, creating tension throughout the whole muscle system.

The Liver/Gallbladder System also helps the body detoxify and is very sensitive to toxins. The joints are part of this system and respond very quickly to the presence of toxins in the body. You can easily see the relationship between the joints and the Liver/Gallbladder System when you get the flu: the toxins from the inflammation often cause our joints to ache. Other sources of toxins like medicines and mercury fillings, as well as the bacteria from root canals, also compromise the liver.

As mentioned above, the Liver/Gallbladder System is one of the major systems that control the processes of the reproductive organs. When factors such as birth control pills, IUDs, hormone replacement therapy, hysterectomies, tubal ligations, and vasectomies compromise the reproductive organs, the Liver/Gallbladder System is affected. As a result, chronic muscle pain and diseases such as fibromyalgia can develop.

Other Systems and the Muscles

Like the Liver/Gallbladder System, the Kidney/Bladder System plays a specific role in the functions of muscle tissue. The bladder controls the initial energies of the immune system that flow through the body's muscles and connective tissues, and also supports all muscle groups. Backache, for example, is most often a bladder issue because part of the bladder's energy system runs through the long muscles controlling the spine. Furthermore, the Kidney/Bladder System controls certain aspects of the reproductive organs. The same factors listed above (birth control pills, IUDs, etc.) will create issues in the Kidney/Bladder System and affect the bladder's ability to stabilize muscle functions.

In addition, the Kidney/Bladder System controls the integrity of the bone tissue, the bone marrow, and the nerve tissues of the brain. Health problems with the bones, such as osteoporosis, are mainly due to chronic disturbances of the Kidney/Bladder System. This system is directly connected not only to digestive processes and their energies, but also to the function of the reproductive organs. Not surprisingly, loss of bone tissue often occurs during or after menopause. During menopause, the body demands more of the Kidney/

Bladder System due to the natural changes that are occurring. If the kidneys have not been functioning well previously, or if the reproductive system's functional relationship to the kidneys has been compromised by the use of birth control pills, hysterectomy, IUDs, or hormone replacement therapy, the Kidney/Bladder System will be deficient and unable to nourish the bone tissue.

The Spleen/Stomach System also plays an important role in the health of the muscles. The spleen distributes the primary energies that come from the food we digest. When the spleen and stomach are not functioning well, the muscles do not receive the nourishment they need and become weak.

Movement and Health

Our bodies are made to *move,* so exercise is very important. Keep in mind, however, that over-exercising will compromise the body's structural system. Also, remember that the body moves naturally in *circular* movements—in a rhythm of contraction and relaxation of all muscle groups. Static movements, or exercises that cause muscles only to contract or move in straight lines, like some weight lifting techniques, will build muscle tissue but compromise the integrity of the body's structural system. Likewise, high-impact exercises like jogging and aerobics can overstimulate the central nerve system and compromise both the Kidney/Bladder and Liver/Gallbladder Systems. Swimming, dancing, hiking, and disciplines like T'ai Chi are excellent for the healthy maintenance of the muscle system.

THERAPY

MUSCLE PAIN

General Remedies

Remedy #1

- Fresh castor oil or olive oil
- 2 teaspoons ginger powder
- 1 teaspoon turmeric (if available)

Mix enough warm castor or olive oil with the ginger powder and the turmeric (if you have it). Apply twice a day and/or overnight.

Remedy #2

- Olive Oil

Rub oil on painful area.

Remedy #3
- Epsom salt

Follow directions on the carton to make an Epsom salt bath. Soak for 15–20 minutes once daily.

Spices and Herbs

- **Black pepper**

  PREPARATION METHOD: Herbal oil; include in the daily diet
- **Cayenne pepper**

  PREPARATION METHOD: Herbal oil; include in the daily diet
- **Cinnamon**

  PREPARATION METHOD: Standard hot infusion, dry plant tincture, herbal oil, herbal bath
- **Garlic**

  PREPARATION METHOD: Fresh plant tincture, dry plant tincture, herbal compress, herbal oil
- **Oregano**

  PREPARATION METHOD: Standard hot infusion, fresh plant tincture, dry plant tincture, herbal oil, herbal bath
- **Thyme and rosemary**

  PREPARATION METHOD: Decoction, fresh plant tincture, dry plant tincture, herbal oil, herbal bath

Foods

- **Asparagus**

  PREPARATION METHOD: Vegetable compress
- **Carrots**

  PREPARATION METHOD: Vegetable compress
- **Castor oil pack**

  PREPARATION METHOD: Soak a wool or plain cotton cloth in warm castor oil. Place on site of discomfort and cover with a piece of plastic wrap. Next, cover this with a towel and place a hot water bottle on the site (or use without) and wrap into place. Do not use a heating pad.
- **Celery**

  PREPARATION METHOD: See Detox for the Digestive Tract and Joints, page 200.
- **Lemon**

  PREPARATION METHOD: Fruit compress, fruit juice application
- **Oats**

  PREPARATION METHOD: Compress, herbal bath

- **Olive pits**

   PREPARATION METHOD: Crush one dried olive pit and drink with a little water 1–2 times a day; dry plant tincture; herbal oil
- **Onion**

   PREPARATION METHOD: Make a compress with diced raw onions and one teaspoon of salt; fresh plant tincture
- **Potato**

   PREPARATION METHOD: Make a mashed-potato compress and place on site.

SORE BACK MUSCLES

Tissue Salts

- *Calc. phos. 6X*
- *Mag. phos. 6X*
- *Natrum sulph. 6X*
- *Kali sulph. 6X*
- *Calc. fluor. 6X*

   Take these remedies together 3–4 times daily for up to three days. Then reduce the number of doses to 2–3 times daily for up to one additional week, if necessary. Reduce the number of doses as symptoms begin to improve.

WEAKNESS OF DISCS

Tissue Salts

- *Calc. fluor. 6X*
- *Calc. phos. 6X*
- *Kali phos. 6X*

   Take these remedies together twice daily for three weeks. Reduce the number of doses as symptoms begin to improve.

ARTHRITIC PAINS

General Remedies

Remedy #1
- Cabbage leaves

   Take 2 large (juicy, not dry) cabbage leaves and place them in a pot of rapidly boiling water for 1 minute or until they are a little floppy. Remove and let cool a little, then apply them directly to the area of pain for $1/2$ hour. Hold them in place with a wrung-out towel that has been soaked in the water used to soften the leaves. This can be repeated several times a day.

Remedy #2
- Castor oil

Apply warm, fresh castor oil in a compress to the affected area. This can be done several times a day.

Remedy #3
- 6 teaspoons ginger powder
- 6 teaspoons ground caraway seeds
- 3 teaspoons ground black pepper

Mix ginger powder, caraway seeds, and black pepper together. Take $\frac{1}{2}$ teaspoon of this mixture with water two times per day.

Tissue Salts
- *Natrum mur.* 6X
- *Natrum sulph.* 6X
- *Natrum phos.* 6X

Take 3–4 times daily for up to six days. Reduce the number of doses as symptoms begin to improve.

Spices, Herbs, and Foods
- **Garlic**

  PREPARATION METHOD: Fresh plant tincture, dry plant tincture, herbal compress, herbal oil
- **Ginger**

  PREPARATION METHOD: Herbal compress, herbal oil, herbal bath
- **Asparagus**

  PREPARATION METHOD: Vegetable compress
- **Castor oil packs**

  PREPARATION METHOD: Soak a wool or plain cotton cloth in warm castor oil. Place on the site of discomfort and cover with a piece of plastic wrap. Next, cover this with a towel and place a hot water bottle on top (or use without) and wrap into place. Do not use a heating pad.
- **Celery**

  PREPARATION METHOD: See Detox for the Digestive Tract and Joints on page 200.
- **Honey/apple cider vinegar**

  PREPARATION METHOD: Add 1 teaspoon of honey and 1 teaspoon of apple cider vinegar to a glass of water. Drink 1–2 times per day.
- **Lemon**

  PREPARATION METHOD: Fruit compress, fruit juice application

- **Potato**

PREPARATION METHOD: Make a mashed-potato compress and place on site.

Detox for the Digestive Tract and Joints:

Place 1 cup raw spinach and 1 cup apple juice in a blender. Drink 1–2 cups daily; if available, 1 hour after drinking the mixture, drink 1 cup of celery juice followed an hour later by 1 cup of carrot juice.

SWELLING

General Remedies

Remedy #1

- Barley

Mix 1 part barley with 4 parts water. In a pan with the lid on, boil gently for 20 minutes. Strain and drink one cup 2–3 times per day.

Remedy #2

- Coriander

Make a tea by adding 1 teaspoon of coriander powder to 1 cup of boiling water. Drink 2 cups daily.

Remedy #3

- Salt
- Turmeric
- Castor oil or olive oil

Mix 1 part salt to 2 parts turmeric. Add enough fresh castor oil or olive oil to make a paste. Apply to area as a compress.

Tissue Salts

- *Kali mur.* 6X
- *Natrum mur.* 6X
- *Natrum sulph.* 6X

Take these remedies together 3–4 times daily for up to 6 days. Reduce the number of doses as symptoms begin to improve.

GENERAL CARE OF MUSCLES AND JOINTS

Spices and Herbs

- **Basil**

THERAPEUTIC ACTION: Relieves feeling of numbness

PREPARATION METHOD: Standard hot infusion, fresh plant tincture, dry plant tincture, herbal compress, herbal oil, herbal bath

- **Black pepper**
  THERAPEUTIC ACTION: Relieves backache, neuralgia, and rheumatism
  PREPARATION METHOD: Herbal oil; include in the daily diet
- **Cayenne pepper**
  THERAPEUTIC ACTION: Relieves muscle pain, backache, and neuritis
  PREPARATION METHOD: Herbal oil; include in the daily diet
- **Chicory**
  THERAPEUTIC ACTION: Relieves painful joints and rheumatism
  PREPARATION METHOD: Standard hot infusion, fresh plant tincture, herbal compress, herbal oil
- **Cinnamon**
  THERAPEUTIC ACTION: Relieves neuralgia, rheumatism, myalgia, and cramps
  PREPARATION METHOD: Standard hot infusion, dry plant tincture, herbal oil, herbal bath
- **Garlic**
  THERAPEUTIC ACTION: Relieves rheumatism and arthritis pain
  PREPARATION METHOD: Fresh plant tincture, dry plant tincture, herbal compress, herbal oil
- **Ginger**
  THERAPEUTIC ACTION: Relieves arthritis
  PREPARATION METHOD: Herbal compress, herbal oil, herbal bath
- **Oregano**
  THERAPEUTIC ACTION: Relieves rheumatism in muscles and joints
  PREPARATION METHOD: Standard hot infusion, fresh plant tincture, dry plant tincture, herbal oil, herbal bath
- **Thyme and rosemary**
  THERAPEUTIC ACTION: Relieves acute neuralgia and muscle pain
  PREPARATION METHOD: Decoction, fresh plant tincture, dry plant, herbal oil, herbal bath
- **Turmeric**
  THERAPEUTIC ACTION: Relieves arthritic and rheumatic pain and sprains
  PREPARATION METHOD: Mix lime juice with turmeric powder until slightly runny and use as a compress; fresh plant tincture, herbal oil, herbal bath

Foods

- **Asparagus**
  THERAPEUTIC ACTION: Relieves numb limbs, muscle spasm and twitching, stiff tendons, lower back pain, rheumatism, and arthritis
  PREPARATION METHOD: Vegetable compress

- **Castor oil packs**

  THERAPEUTIC ACTION: Relieves joint and muscle pain

  PREPARATION METHOD: Soak a wool or plain cotton cloth in warm castor oil. Place on the site of discomfort and cover with a piece of plastic wrap. Next, cover this with a towel and place a hot water bottle on top (or use without) and wrap into place. Do not use a heating pad.

- **Carrots**

  THERAPEUTIC ACTION: Relieves rheumatism pain

  PREPARATION METHOD: Vegetable compress

- **Green tea**

  THERAPEUTIC ACTION: Relieves arthritis

  PREPARATION METHOD: Wet a tea bag and place on site of discomfort; dry plant tincture

- **Honey and apple cider vinegar**

  THERAPEUTIC ACTION: Relieves joint pain and reduces gouty deposits in joints

  PREPARATION METHOD: Add 1 teaspoon of honey and 1 teaspoon of apple cider vinegar to a glass of water. Drink 1–2 times per day.

- **Lemon**

  THERAPEUTIC ACTION: Relieves arthritis and rheumatism

  PREPARATION METHOD: Fruit compress, fruit juice application

- **Oats**

  THERAPEUTIC ACTION: Relieves neuralgia, sciatica, and rheumatism

  PREPARATION METHOD: Compress, herbal bath

- **Olive pits**

  THERAPEUTIC ACTION: Relieves backache

  PREPARATION METHOD: Crush 1 dried olive pit and drink with a little water 1–2 times a day; dry plant tincture; herbal oil

- **Onions**

  THERAPEUTIC ACTION: Relieves sprains and bruises

  PREPARATION METHOD: Make a compress with $1/2$ cup diced raw onion mixed with 1 teaspoon of salt; fresh plant tincture

- **Potato**

  THERAPEUTIC ACTION: Relieves aches, pains, and inflammation in joints and muscles

  PREPARATION METHOD: Make a mashed-potato compress and place on the site of discomfort

> **Detox for the Digestive Tract and Joints:** Place 1 part raw spinach and 1 part apple juice in a blender. Drink 1–2 glasses daily; 1 hour after

drinking the mixture, drink 1 cup of celery juice followed 1 hour later by 1 cup of carrot juice (if these juices are available).

Reflexology

For instructions on reflexology, see "Reflexology" under "How to Use the Therapy Section" at the beginning of Part II.

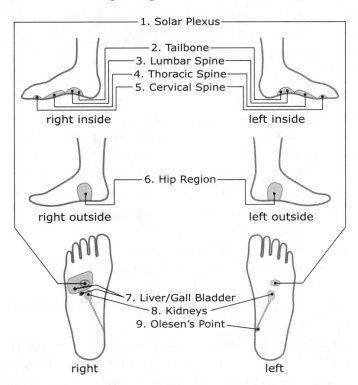

PAIN

TEACHING

Pain is one of the important communication systems of the body and mind. Like the other senses, it makes us aware of vital issues to which the body is responding. All tissues contain a nerve system. These sensitive nerves tell us what is going on in particular tissues by sending messages to the brain. If a tissue is compromised by trauma or is responding to part of its healing process, the brain returns a signal to the tissue and pain occurs.

The pain produced by most healing processes in tissues is a result of swelling and heightened metabolism in the tissue. The swelling is due to extra fluids that are created around compromised tissues. These fluids are an important part of the healing process and contain immune substances as well as nutrients that nourish and build up the compromised cells.

Compromised tissues can also become inflamed. The inflammation is not the disease or the trauma itself, but a way that the body heals itself by elevating the metabolism of the tissue in order to support its cells and ensure their survival and well-being.

Psychological Aspects of Pain

One of the important, yet often overlooked, aspects of pain is the psychological component. Pain itself is a purely physical phenomenon caused by the factors mentioned above. When we "hurt," however, our psyche immediately tries to interpret what is happening to us. It brings into this interpretation an acute sense that something is threatening our person. This sense of threat involves all the conscious and unconscious memories—or programs—that the psyche has created in the past. If these memories involve feelings of insecurity, loneliness, and vulnerability, we become anxious and perhaps fearful. This reaction creates tension in the body, further increasing the pain and decreasing our ability to integrate it.

We never experience physical pain alone because our psyches are participating in everything that happens to us. Rather, we "suffer" with pain because we have a hard time stopping the psyche from telling us that we are in trouble and that the situation might be out of control. We feel vulnerable and threatened by the feeling of pain, but the psyche cannot interpret accurately what's really happening on a cellular and tissue level. It's as though a red warning light has gone on in your car and you don't know if you just need more oil or if the motor is damaged.

Dealing with this aspect of pain can be difficult. Remember when you're in pain that you're only *experiencing* pain: that pain is a physical reaction of the body doing what it knows best, which includes sending itself important messages, determining what has to be done, and starting the healing process. Try to be calm and allow the body to get on with that process.

Because the psyche is so involved, pain can affect our quality of life. During periods of severe pain, it can be appropriate to use chemical drugs such as painkillers to alleviate the pain. These drugs, of course, have side effects, so they should be used in limited dosages and for the shortest time possible.

Never take painkillers to completely eradicate pain; use only enough to make the pain tolerable. Even nonprescription drugs like aspirin have side effects that will severely interfere with the body's processes. Taking aspirin, for instance, to alleviate chronic headaches or joint pain is not a good idea. Consult a natural healthcare professional and cure the cause of the pain in a natural way.

THERAPY

Spices and Herbs

All of the substances listed below can be used to help relieve pain in any part of the body.

- **Clove**
  PREPARATION METHOD: Decoction (use as a compress), dry plant tincture, herbal oil, herbal bath
- **Garlic**
  PREPARATION METHOD: Fresh plant tincture, herbal compress, herbal oil, garlic oil
- **Ginger**
  PREPARATION METHOD: Standard hot infusion, standard cold infusion, fresh plant tincture, dry plant tincture, herbal compress, herbal oil, herbal wine, herbal bath

Foods

- **Almonds**
  PREPARATION METHOD: Herbal wine; include in the diet
- **Apples**
  PREPARATION METHOD: Fruit compress; include in the diet
- **Black or green tea**
  PREPARATION METHOD: Compress using tea bag wetted with water
- **Castor oil**
  PREPARATION METHOD: Use fresh castor oil. Soak a small clean cloth in warmed oil and place on the painful area. After opening, always store oil in refrigerator.
- **Chili peppers**
  PREPARATION METHOD: Crush chili peppers (or use powdered cayenne pepper) and mix into a paste with olive oil; apply to site of discomfort.
- **Dried dates**
  PREPARATION METHOD: Fruit compress; include in the diet

- **Gherkins (small pickles)**
  PREPARATION METHOD: Vegetable compress
- **Onion**
  PREPARATION METHOD: Fresh plant tincture
- **Oranges**
  PREPARATION METHOD: Fruit compress; include in the daily diet
- **Pineapples**
  PREPARATION METHOD: Fruit compress
- **Prunes**
  PREPARATION METHOD: Fruit compress
- **Sugar (pure cane)**
  PREPARATION METHOD: Wet sugar with water and place directly on painful site; hold in place with a cloth.
- **Sweet peppers**
  PREPARATION METHOD: Vegetable compress

Reflexology

For instructions on reflexology, see "Reflexology" under "How to Use the Therapy Section" at the beginning of Part II.

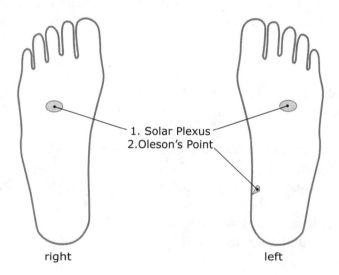

1. Solar Plexus
2. Oleson's Point

right   left

PREGNANCY AND BIRTH

TEACHING

Life is a sacred system of simple principles and infinitely complex relation-ships. Beginning in the late 1500s, the sciences of Western culture began to distinguish between "living" and "non-living" entities: a human being, grass, animals, and plants are living, whereas rocks and water are nonliving. The sciences of other cultures, however, have always considered the whole uni-verse and everything in it as living. They see everything as sharing the "liv-ingness" of all life. In other words, everything builds, maintains, grows, and changes within the same set of universal principles and mechanisms.

Modern research, particularly in the area of quantum physics, has shown that it is inaccurate to divide life into living and nonliving systems because all things that exist interact with and are intimately connected with one another. Even soil, rocks, and water have mechanisms of sensitivity and growth just as the human body does, but each in their own way. To understand the human body and mind, we must see ourselves as part of and sharing a cosmic envi-ronment. The life that moves within our bodies through our blood, cells, and tissues is connected *directly* to the most distant star systems as well as the immediate environment surrounding us.

Thus, our bodies really have no "inside" and "outside": the air we breathe, the water we drink, and the food we eat are made up of the elements from the life energies of the nature "outside" of us to the universe beyond. Yet, these energies become the chemistry, cells, and tissues of our bodies. This sharing of substances, events, and energies becomes apparent when we consider that the fetal child grows and develops even as we do—by taking in the nutrients and energies from the world of life around him or her.

The Soil for New Life

Conception is most easily understood through the following analogy. The female egg (ovum) is like the seed of a plant. When we plant a seed in soil, water it, and care for it, a plant grows. That tiny seed contains all the elements and energies of the plant. Similarly, the ovum when fertilized contains the entire being of the new child including the codes and primary life energies that will further develop this unique human being, just as miraculously as a plant appears when we sow a seed in the fertilizing earth. The male sperm is like the sun and water—it contains the energies to open and fertilize the seed so that it can begin its development from seed to plant. The mother's body becomes the soil through which the fertilized seed grows to its fullness, ready for birth.

In our modern culture, there have been many scientific debates as to when a fertilized egg and its developing fetus becomes human. Some say that a human being is present only after three months, some say after six months, and so on. This debate, of course, is all quite ridiculous. Just as the seed contains the entire "plant" replete with all the mechanisms of heredity and life energies that characterize its living and emerging being, so the egg fertilized by the sperm contains the whole individual from the very moment of conception. We do not become more of a true human being over time; we're *conceived* that way. The only thing that happens over time is that we develop the potentials that are already present at this sacred moment of conception.

At the moment of conception, two things happen: a new human being emerges in the universe of creation and the mother's body changes totally as she becomes the environment of new life. This concept of fetal environment is seen throughout nature. A bird's egg, for example, serves as the environment for the developing avian fetus. In most species, the mother bird changes her usual activities in order to constantly protect the egg and provide a suitable nest for the life of the developing fetus. In humans and animals, the fetus grows and develops within the mother's body. Hence, her body becomes the natural environment of the fetal child's world, the nest for new life.

Becoming the environment for new life during pregnancy impacts the mother enormously. The new individual, now the fetal child, is an inseparable part of her bodily functions and mental and emotional experiences. Becoming pregnant is a profound change that affects the body's biochemistry, cells, and tissues, and initiates the intimate communication of thoughts and feelings between the mother and child.

We often think of the mind as being private and that only our spoken words or our outward behavior convey what we're thinking or feeling. This perception is inaccurate. Our mind formulates thoughts that may never become words and feelings that may never be expressed. Nevertheless, these thoughts and feelings clearly speak to the fetal child. Likewise, the fetal child can communicate its consciousness of relationship and its feelings with the mother.

Because of these profound changes that take place at conception and throughout the development of the fetal child, miscarriages and abortions also strongly influence the mother. We can imagine the total change that has been taking place since conception and the deep communication that is part of this relationship between the mother and the fetal child suddenly ending. Even when, in the case of abortion, the parents are in agreement about the reason to terminate the pregnancy, and as much sense as their reasons seem to make, the abrupt ending of life and its relationship to the mother's own body and psyche have a very powerful effect. It takes a long time for the mother's body and mind to adjust to the situation and resume her life without the other. Often, a remnant of sorrow lingers on very deep unconscious levels. The psyche may have difficulty resolving the event even when other parts of the mind are reconciled to the decision.

Development of the Fetal Child

As previously discussed, all cells, tissues, and organ systems of our bodies develop from one of three original embryological tissues. The mesoderm embryological tissue produces the body's connective tissue, bones, cartilage, muscles, blood cells, lymph, spleen, kidneys, heart, reproductive organs, and blood vessels. The mesoderm represents the integration system of the mind and body. It mediates between the ectoderm and endoderm systems, helping them to work well together, and is the psychological vehicle for our growing consciousness and spirituality.

The ectoderm embryological tissue produces the skin, nails, nerve tissue, and brain. This is the body's communication system. Psychologically, the ectoderm system responds to "territorial" events that occur in the environment around us. Conflicts at home, at work, or in school, for instance, will affect the tissues and functions of this system.

The endoderm embryological tissue produces the digestive organs and glands. This is the "nutrition" system. Psychologically, the endoderm system responds to our need for nutrients and the ability to process them. Our nutritional needs are not confined just to the food we eat, but also include our need to be nourished emotionally, mentally, and spiritually. Not receiving the proper nutrition in any of these areas will affect the organs of the endoderm system.

We must not forget that the three tissue systems and their physical organs and psychological processes function in the same way in the fetal child as in the full-born child. Thus, we can see that the fetal child has a full and active life that functions exactly as ours does. Caring for the fetal child is no different from caring for ourselves. Providing the right nutrition for the mother, creating a peaceful and supporting environment around the expecting mother, and consciously communicating with the fetal child are all essential components in the life phases of pregnancy.

THERAPY

MORNING SICKNESS

Due to the profound changes that occur in the mother's body after conception, certain symptoms like morning sickness can arise. This is caused by the formation of new functional patterns in the mother's systems that accommodate the fetal child.

Tissue Salts

- *Kali mur. 6X*
- *Natrum mur. 6X*
- *Natrum phos. 6X*

Take these remedies together 3 times daily for up to three weeks. Reduce the number of doses as symptoms begin to improve.

Spices, Herbs, and Foods

- **Cinnamon**

  PREPARATION METHOD: Standard hot infusion, dry plant tincture, herbal bath
- **Ginger**

  PREPARATION METHOD: Standard hot infusion, fresh plant tincture, dry plant tincture

GENERAL SUPPORT DURING PREGNANCY

Spices, Herbs, and Foods

- **Sage**

  THERAPEUTIC ACTION: Internal antibiotic

  PREPARATION METHOD: Standard hot infusion, fresh plant tincture, dry plant tincture, herbal bath
- **Corn silk (the silk around the cob)**

  THERAPEUTIC ACTION: Helps pass urine; reduces swelling of ankles, feet, and tissues during pregnancy

  PREPARATION METHOD: Simmer a large handful of corn silk in 1 quart of water for 10 minutes. Drink 1–2 glasses of liquid per day for up to three weeks.
- **Egg shells**

  THERAPEUTIC ACTION: Builds calcium during pregnancy

  PREPARATION METHOD: Clean and dry several organic egg shells. Boil the shells for 3 minutes, then remove from the water and dry. Crush the shells into a powder. Add $\frac{1}{2}$ teaspoon of powder to food.

SUPPORT FOR NURSING

Spices, Herbs, and Foods

- **Anise seed**
  THERAPEUTIC ACTION: Promotes breast milk
  PREPARATION METHOD: Standard hot infusion, dry plant tincture, herbal bath
- **Caraway**
  THERAPEUTIC ACTION: Promotes flow of milk
  PREPARATION METHOD: Standard hot infusion, dry plant tincture, herbal bath
- **Celery**
  THERAPEUTIC ACTION: Promotes breast milk
  PREPARATION METHOD: Vegetable compress
- **Fennel seed**
  THERAPEUTIC ACTION: Promotes lactation; benefits functions of breasts; relieves engorged breasts; reduces breast lumps; relieves symptom of curdled breast milk (*Note: Do not use during pregnancy*)
  PREPARATION METHOD: Decoction, dry plant tincture, vegetable compress (to make compress, boil fennel seed with an equal part of barley; use 1–3 times daily)
- **Fenugreek seed**
  THERAPEUTIC ACTION: Increases milk
  PREPARATION METHOD: Standard hot infusion, dry plant tincture, herbal oil, herbal bath
- **Parsley**
  THERAPEUTIC ACTION: Softens hard breasts in early stage of nursing
  PREPARATION METHOD: Herbal compress

PSYCHOLOGICAL ISSUES

TEACHING

In allopathic medicine, the mind has remained a mystery and no suitable models have been developed to describe its function. Doctors and psychiatrists have found certain chemical aspects of brain functions that have an impact on emotional and psychological responses. As a result, the field of psychiatry tends to focus primarily on the chemical mechanisms that influence our emotions and moods. It relies on chemical drugs to treat conditions like anxiety and depression. These medicines all have two things in common:

they all have major side effects and they do not correct or resolve the true problem, but rather alter the chemistry of the body, masking the symptoms. Remember that a symptom like anxiety, for example, is a *symptom* of an underlying *cause*, it is not a cause itself. Without resolving the cause, there is no real healing.

Symptoms like depression and anxiety are very uncomfortable and it is understandable that one will mistake the masking of the symptom through chemical intervention as being a "cure," but the opposite is actually the case. Unless the causes of the symptom are resolved, the essential factors will only be suppressed; true resolution will not occur. The chemistry involved in brain functions (like all other chemical reactions in the body) is created by the function of the body's tissues and organ systems. These functions are affected by both emotional stress factors as well as by physiological factors like toxins, lifestyle, and surgery, and by chemical drugs that influence the body's chemistry. Drugs only deal with the superficial symptoms and do not change or heal the causes of the faulty chemistry.

The Unity of Body and Mind

For centuries, Classical medicine has used clear, functional models to better understand the mind and how to treat it. One of the major contributions has been in understanding that the psyche, the emotional aspect of the mind, is in reality controlled by the major organ systems of the body. In other words, our emotional responses are not so much determined by any particular situation but by the body's ability to "digest," process, and integrate our emotional and mental experiences through the metabolic mechanisms inherent in the body's organs.

Classical medical traditions have taught us that our ability to process what we are experiencing is dependent on the functions of our major organ and tissue systems. They recognize that the Liver/Gallbladder System controls the emotions of angst, hate, irritation, anger, and jealousy; the Kidney/Bladder System controls feelings of fear and anxiety; the Stomach/Spleen System controls feelings of worry and obsessive behavior; the Colon/Lung System controls the feelings of grief and "stress"; and the Heart/Small Intestine System controls the feeling of well-being and integration as well as the sense of self.

Our emotions and the emotional part of our mind reflect the function of our organ systems. The mind and the body are not two different things, but *a unified whole*. We can see this clearly in the practice of acupuncture. This therapy uses a needle to penetrate energy points that directly affect an organ system's function. When done correctly, an acupuncturist can successfully treat anxiety disorders, depression, and schizophrenia, for example, without any form of drugs or psychotherapy, simply by balancing the functional energies of the organ systems that control these patterns and responses. In this sense, natural medical practices recognize that psychological symptoms are most often caused by chronic functional disturbances in the body, rather than in the mind. Emotions, therefore, are *symptoms*, not causes of "emotional disorders."

The immune system plays an important role in mental health as well. As you recall, the immune system is not a defense system but an integration system. It not only helps us to live in harmony with our physical surroundings but also helps us integrate our mental and emotional life with our environment. Therefore, any form of psychotherapy must respect and be sensitive to the integration processes of the immune system that are taking place on an emotional level within the individual. The immune system will repress events that are too traumatic to deal with, until a time when we are able to integrate them. Forcing the mind to resolve issues that it is unprepared for can lead to deeper psychological imbalances and further health problems. An essential part of this preparation is ensuring that the organ systems that regulate the emotions are functioning well, providing a solid foundation for working with our emotions.

The Emotions and Our Psyche

Psychiatrists and psychologists often use past experiences as the point of reference for helping a person cope with their mental and emotional issues. This approach can be helpful because when we communicate the details of our past, we are able to re-examine our experiences and responses. Communicating these patterns with another person can bring new clarity and perspective into the way we react to life situations. We all need some form of positive, supportive feedback. Others can help us toward understanding ourselves better as well as comforting us when emotional stresses become overwhelming. As positive as psychological care and counseling can be, it often overlooks the fact that most psychological issues are due to disturbances in the body's functional systems.

Emotions are a vital part of human life and serve to inspire us, help us grow and mature, and orient us to the social aspects of our nature and personality. "Negative" emotions do not exist. *All* emotions are part of the wonderful kaleidoscope of human responses, which contribute to our lives through the experiencing of them, no matter how hard they are to deal with. Society tends to divide emotions into good (happiness, contentment, inspiration, etc.) and bad (anger, anxiety, depression, etc.). We are supposed to suppress or eliminate the bad emotions and only respond to the good ones. This perspective, of course, is completely neurotic in itself—it is bad for our mental health and creates a false picture of the world and our responses to living as unique individuals within a collective environment.

A major contribution of Classical medicine is in distinguishing between the psyche and its emotional content and consciousness, the spiritual dimension. The psyche relates to organ system functions and it creates the immediate sense of who we are in the ever-changing environment of events that we experience in daily life. The psyche functions on the level of emotional responses, which are controlled by the ability of the body's organ systems to process and integrate our experiences. The psyche is also involved in our ability to process knowledge and to learn new skills. The psyche is the organ of our identity; it brings forth the visible features of who we think we are, while clothing the mystery of Self.

Consciousness and Spirituality

The consciousness is a deeper dimension of the person and has always been associated with the inner authentic self. Our consciousness is not so much a matter of who we think we are as it is of who we *really* are. Increasing our understanding of who we truly are is the very foundation of all spiritual traditions and religions. The psychological dimension of our mind interprets things directly from our experiences. It sorts experiences into bad ones to be avoided and good ones to grasp on to. The psyche is not capable of dealing with the ultimate nature of an experience or what the ultimate meaning of an experience is, beyond it being pleasurable or not.

Emotions play an important role in what makes us human and they are the vehicle for our motivations and creative abilities. In this sense, emotions relate to our deeper spiritual nature as well as to the physical functions of the body. To understand the true nature of emotions, therefore, we must examine their spiritual side.

Chinese medicine has provided us with a concise and insightful understanding of the vital interface between the spirit and the body/mind functions, including the emotions. The foundation of all aspects of the human being is the spirit with its universal consciousness. The spirit penetrates the body/mind at the level of the five main organ systems. Each organ system has its own particular connection to the working of the spirit within its own functional framework. In Chinese medicine, each system is defined by its particular "spirit" or fundamental motivation, which facilitates and governs its functions in the overall mind/body/spirit connection. We will use the original Chinese terms for the organ system "spirits" to avoid confusion along with a short description of each system.

The Heart System is the master spirit called *shen*, overseeing all of the other mind/body/spirit connections. It is the vital center of the human being and makes the direct connection between the individual and the universal nature of the spirit possible. It provides the rhythm and balance among all systems and their activities—spiritual, mental, emotional, and physical.

The connection with the Liver System and the spirit is called *hun* and is the first of the organ systems to begin programming the mind/body functions. *Hun* translates as "the imager." The *hun* facilitates the imprinting of personal hereditary energies from the individual's gene pool that stem from the patterns of the Kidney System and, by way of these patterns, form all the other organ system energies into our constitution. *Hun* also carries the "image and likeness of God" that connects us to the sacredness of all creation and the divine presence, bringing our spiritual activities into the body and mind.

The Lung System's "spirit" is called *po* and provides the vital energy for being, growth, and personal development. It carries the cosmic energies that activate and run the patterns created by the Liver System's "spirit" *hun*. The lungs' *po* is our connection to the universal creative forces of life that pervade the entire cosmos.

The Kidney System's "spirit" is *zhi*. *Zhi* forms the intentionality of the human mind and body. It is the inner will and wisdom to live and function found within all cells and tissues. *Zhi* is also the psychic authority that moves the organism to the realization of all its potentials. It provides the lungs' *po* with the will to be and the skills of body and mind to achieve the fullness of life.

The Spleen System's "spirit" is called *yi*. *Yi* is the functional interface between the body and mind. It integrates all the other systems' "spirits" with the body's organ and tissue functions and creates the connection between the emotions and the physical body. *Yi* helps us access our deeper consciousness and regulates the mental and physical dispositions that determine our behavior.

The spirit's deep consciousness reflects only the beauty and truth of reality, which is beyond any functional disturbances of the body or the psyche's ability to harmonize the circumstances of our lives. Ultimately, the ability to emote is connected to positive, life-affirming, and life-giving qualities. These qualities reflect the eternal good that makes up the spirit and is always at work within our bodies and mind. This goodness can be hard to recognize when we are experiencing "negative" emotions. To understand the spiritual aspect of negative emotions, we need to look closer at the deeper foundations of emotions themselves.

The spirit is like a mirror that only reflects reality, which is the eternal goodness and beauty of life. When this image of life is reflected through the prism of the body and psyche, however, it can become distorted and create what we call negative emotions. In reality, we are only capable of producing *positive* emotions, but functional disturbances in our organ systems that affect the psyche, as well as lack of conscious contact with our spirituality, can distort the positive emotional image from the deep consciousness of our spirit. In other words, negative emotions are really only *distortions* of true, positive emotions.

To become emotionally healthy, we need to understand how negative emotions conceal positive ones. Every emotion has two sides—one is the true positive side, and the other is the distortion. It is important to understand that in every emotional experience these two sides are present simultaneously.

There are four basic categories of negative emotions that we experience at one time or another. The first is fear. Fear is a response to anything we perceive as a threat, from a physical attack to more vague and anxious feelings about the dangers that seem to be lurking in life. It would be impossible to feel fear if we did not have something positive that could be threatened. The positive, true emotions behind the negative distortion of fear are faith, confidence, love, and being loved unconditionally.

A second negative emotion is inappropriate desire, which has nothing to do with positive expectations but is connected to distorted feelings of self-worth. Inappropriate desire tells us that we need to be more beautiful and smarter, more skillful and successful, or have more money, position, and respect in order to feel happy and fulfilled. In the background of this distorted emotion of unworthiness is the true and positive reality of being loved and being worthy of love without any conditions.

Anger, envy, and jealousy are negative emotions that are imbedded in one another. We experience these distorted emotions when we feel that someone has something we don't have, is going to take something from us, or that life doesn't seem to support us in the way we need to be supported. Perhaps someone has a different belief or opinion that angers us. Perhaps someone takes what we feel is ours or owns something that we think we should have, leaving us feeling jealous. When these distorted emotions become chronic, they will ultimately result in depression, a state during which we experience that we can't control the actions of others for our own benefit. Behind these distortions is the positive emotion of compassion, an understanding and unconditional acceptance of another, which is grounded in the reality of true love. Compassion desires the best for every person and responds by loving them in spite of what they do or have.

One overlooked negative emotion is ignorance. In this respect, ignorance does not mean how intelligent we are or how much we know, but refers to *willful* ignorance—the unwillingness to hear, see, or acknowledge anything that threatens our entrenched positions regarding life and how to live it. Willful ignorance effectively stops our ability to mature intellectually, emotionally, and spiritually by resisting change and personal growth. We resist the changes that new ideas bring into our lives and stubbornly hold onto our old positions, unwilling to let them develop and evolve. The positive emotion in the background of willful ignorance is openness and clarity. It is through these emotions, which envelop awe and wonder, that our minds and bodies experience the deepest connectedness to life. The clarity of reality reflects love and beauty like a mirror into our very beings.

It's not enough just to be informed about the nature of our emotions; we need to give attention to them and practice ways of responding to them. It is not the emotion itself or having emotions that are the problem—it is what the emotion reveals to us and how we respond that makes the difference. Many people feel that they have to "heal" negative emotions, that through concerted effort they will be able to eliminate negative emotions and only experience "good" emotions. This, of course, is not possible. As we've seen, negative emotions don't really exist in and of themselves, but are always distortions of positive, life-affirming emotions. We can't eliminate negative emotions, but we can allow ourselves to discover the beauty and goodness of their foundation.

Negative emotions are like clouds covering up the sun. The sun is always there, shining behind the clouds and it's not so much a matter of "moving" the clouds as it is of remembering our contact with the sun behind them. Even when there are clouds, the sun's life-giving energies invisibly penetrate the cloud cover and support the life of the Earth.

It is very difficult to suddenly turn an emotion from its negative manifestation to its positive side when we are in the midst of a powerful emotional experience. If we become angry, for example, we can wait until we have regained a modicum of composure and then recall our anger in a more neutral circumstance. As we remember the experience of anger, we should not feed it nor suppress it but just let it show itself to us with all of its rationalizations and all the things that it's trying to convince us of. Soon it will run out of steam and quiet down. Then we can look for the compassion and understanding of others that is hidden in the anger itself. Sometimes we want to hold onto and support a negative emotion like anger—this is willful ignorance, which blocks our possibilities of being liberated from anger and experiencing life-affirming foundations.

The Buddhist traditions have an interesting way of illustrating the nature of our psychology and negative emotions. One of their oldest teaching tools consists of paintings that show different aspects of the Buddha. The Buddha who is known as the "Compassionate One" is usually pictured in poses of serene and peaceful contemplation. There are, however, paintings that depict frightening, distorted monsters, usually surrounded by fire, standing on corpses or bones and carrying weapons. These are called "the Wrathful Buddhas" and represent negative attitudes and emotions. The point of these illustrated teachings is that the "monster" is in reality Buddha himself; the monster image is a *distortion* of the only true reality, the clarity and compassion of the Buddha. If we could see through the distortions of our emotions, we would see the monster dissolve into the serene and peaceful Buddha once again.

The spiritual dimension of our mind deals with the *meaning* of life, not just how we experience life through our emotions. It deals with the enormous questions of life like death, the meaning of love, our relationship to the world around us, and who we ultimately are beyond what we think or experience. Whether we consciously think about these things or not, they are always a part of our minds and run in the background of our psyche. If we don't address them consciously, they become issues that put pressure on the way we experience life emotionally and limit or distort our emotional responses.

Essentially, spirituality governs the attitudes and perspectives we have concerning life, whereas our emotions are *responses* to these attitudes. Since emotional responses are connected to organ system functions, the spirituality reflecting our attitudes about life also has a direct effect on the body's functions. Our emotions are determined by the energetic and physiological functions of our organ systems as well as by our spiritual perspectives and, together, these factors determine how we look at life.

Fear, for example, is a response to functional issues in the Kidney System as well as a lack of maturity in our spirituality. We could say that the absence of spiritual maturity allows the psyche to perceive the world as being essentially dangerous and threatening. This is an unconscious attitude that can only be overcome by growing and maturing in our spirituality, which acknowledges that life is essentially supportive, loving, and eternally affirmed.

Developing our own spirituality helps balance the difference between our emotional responses to life and our attitudes regarding life. When our spirituality is not consciously active, the emotional psyche will tend to control all of our experiences and responses. Some of these will be valid, but they will be limited by their very nature. An example of this is forgiveness. When we feel a threat to our body, our well-being, or personal integrity, our body/psyche responds to this threat through a strategy of flight from the threat or anger and aggression to overcome the threat. Forgiveness is "unnatural" for the body, which is always trying to protect itself. Forgiveness is a *spiritual* quality of the consciousness that can only intervene in the cycle of flight or anger if we allow the always-present wisdom of our spirituality to teach and inform the psyche about the greater truths that are bound into the very deepest levels of our cells and tissues. Even though we are all spiritual and our spirit is whole and complete within us, we need to consciously access and utilize its tremendous potentials in order for it to be an active influence in our lives and health.

Science and Spirituality

Today, in a modern world dedicated to technological advancement and emotional individualism, we tend to view spiritual and religious practices as outdated and unscientific, and see societies of the past as being more religious simply because they lacked the scientific knowledge we have today. In a way, we could say that science has become the new religion of the modern worldview, and we turn to its research and technologies for explanations regarding the nature and meaning of life. The problem of relying on science to fulfill the spiritual role in our lives is that scientific methods and techniques are only capable of observing certain aspects of our response to life. For example, science can tell us much about the hormones and nerve responses to love, but can never tell us about the *meaning* or nature of love, or its personal significance in our lives.

We tend to forget that science does not address meaning, nor does it address the awe we experience when confronted with events like conception and birth, the meaning of death, the experience of love, or the creative wonders of beauty. These responses are all spiritual in nature and no amount of research into the mechanisms of these things can ever give them meaning. Without a spiritual sense and understanding of the meaningfulness of these fundamental experiences in our lives, we remain insecure, vulnerable, and emotionally distant, living a restricted and often anxious life.

Maintaining Mental Health

Creating and maintaining a healthy mind and emotional life involves making sure that the body's organ systems are functioning in a healthy manner, and that we have some form of personal spiritual practice that deals consciously with our deeper experience of life itself.

Spiritual practices, regardless of the philosophy or tradition from which they come, are always characterized by a sense of gratefulness, hope, and compassion, both for ourselves and for others. The experience of *true* gratefulness, hope, and compassion, is not dependent on any given circumstance of our lives, but is a natural and unconditional attribute of our consciousness, always present in the depths of the self. It is the spiritual aspect of our consciousness that recognizes the important truth that life is sacred and meaningful. To experience this deeper aspect of our nature, we need to be able to focus "inwards" for a time without the distractions of work, play, or other responsibilities. Traditionally, prayer and meditation have been the vehicles that enable us to do so.

THERAPY

MENTAL HYGIENE

A good exercise for personal mental hygiene is called "sitting." It is very effective yet very simple. Find a place where you can be alone and undisturbed in silence for 15–30 minutes. Sit or lie comfortably and relax your body. Stop consciously thinking about things, planning, or getting involved with memories, yet allow the mind to go where it will. Don't consciously use or control it. When it becomes fixed on something, bring it gently back to silence and become aware of how the mind is usually filled with the noises of thinking and feeling. You will see more clearly the *nature* of the mental and emotional strategies that are part of the makeup of your personality. Yet, you will also sense a self behind all of these thoughts and emotions that is always still and at peace, a self that reflects and embraces all life directly from within.

Discovering these layers of ourselves and how they are all present simultaneously (not just the thinking and feeling mind), we become more connected to the core of our being and expand our ability to experience and respond to our lives.

TO REDUCE ANXIETY

General Remedies
Remedy #1
- 3 charcoal tablets
- 1 glass of red wine

Crush the charcoal tablets (available at most drug stores) into a glass of red wine and drink. For children or those who don't tolerate alcohol, gently simmer wine for a few minutes to remove the alcohol, then add the charcoal tablets. For children from ages five to ten, use 2 tablets.

Tissue Salts

- *Calc. phos.* 6X
- *Kali phos.* 6X
- *Natrum phos.* 6X

Take these remedies together 3–4 times daily for up to 5 days; reduce the number of doses as symptoms begin to improve.

Spices, Herbs, and Foods

- **Anise seeds**
PREPARATION METHOD: Standard hot infusion, decoction, dry plant tincture, herbal wine, herbal bath
- **Celery**
PREPARATION METHOD: Fresh plant tincture
- **Marjoram**
PREPARATION METHOD: Standard hot infusion, dry plant tincture, herbal wine, herbal bath
- **Nutmeg**
PREPARATION METHOD: Standard hot infusion, decoction, dry plant tincture, herbal wine, herbal bath
- **Sage**
PREPARATION METHOD: Standard hot infusion, fresh plant tincture, dry plant tincture, herbal wine, herbal bath

TO REDUCE DEPRESSION

General Remedies

Remedy #1
- 1 teaspoon organic apple cider vinegar
- $\frac{1}{3}$ cup of water
- 1 teaspoon of honey

Mix the vinegar with the water. Stir in the honey. Drink in sips 1–2 times daily. This is also good for children's mood swings. Do not use if there is any current tendency to diarrhea.

Remedy #2
- 1 tablespoon lemon juice
- $\frac{1}{2}$ cup of water

- $\frac{1}{2}$ teaspoon cane sugar

Add the lemon juice to the water. Stir in the cane sugar. Drink 2 times per day.

Tissue Salts

- *Calc. fluor.* 6X
- *Calc. sulph.* 6X
- *Kali phos.* 6X
- *Natrum mur.* 6X

Take these remedies together 3–4 times daily for up to 5 days; reduce the number of doses as symptoms begin to improve.

Spices and Herbs

- **Black pepper**

PREPARATION METHOD: Use $\frac{1}{8}$ teaspoon of ground black pepper in food twice daily

- **Cardamom**

PREPARATION METHOD: Standard hot infusion, decoction, dry plant tincture, herbal wine, herbal bath

- **Cayenne pepper**

PREPARATION METHOD: Use $\frac{1}{8}$ teaspoon of powdered cayenne pepper in food twice daily (for adults only)

- **Chicory**

PREPARATION METHOD: Standard hot infusion, decoction, fresh plant tincture, herbal bath

- **Cinnamon**

PREPARATION METHOD: Standard hot infusion, dry plant tincture, herbal wine, herbal bath

- **Cloves**

PREPARATION METHOD: Standard hot infusion, decoction, dry plant tincture, herbal bath

- **Thyme and rosemary**

PREPARATION METHOD: Standard hot infusion, fresh plant tincture, dry plant tincture, herbal bath

Foods

- **Celery**

PREPARATION METHOD: Fresh plant tincture; include celery twice daily in the diet

- **Lettuce**
  PREPARATION METHOD: Decoction, herbal wine; consume with meals twice daily
- **Oats**
  PREPARATION METHOD: Include oatmeal in the diet once or twice daily
- **Pumpkin seeds**
  PREPARATION METHOD: Fresh plant tincture, dry plant tincture; consume $\frac{1}{2}$ cup of raw pumpkin seeds once daily

---

GENERAL CARE OF PSYCHOLOGICAL ISSUES

Spices and Herbs

- **Anise seed**
  THERAPEUTIC ACTION: Relaxes nerves; reduces nervousness and chronic fatigue from overwork or chronic illness
  PREPARATION METHOD: Standard hot infusion, decoction, dry plant tincture, herbal wine, herbal bath
- **Basil**
  THERAPEUTIC ACTION: Reduces nervousness, melancholy, depression, mental and physical exhaustion, shock, and fainting; strengthens adrenal glands; lifts spirits
  PREPARATION METHOD: Standard hot infusion
- **Black pepper**
  THERAPEUTIC ACTION: Stimulates body and mind functions; reduces vertigo
  PREPARATION METHOD: Include in the daily diet
- **Cardamom**
  THERAPEUTIC ACTION: Reduces depression, fatigue, listlessness, and nervous exhaustion; aids memory
  PREPARATION METHOD: Standard hot infusion, decoction, dry plant tincture, herbal wine, herbal bath
- **Cayenne pepper**
  THERAPEUTIC ACTION: Reduces melancholy and depression; acts as a general stimulant
  PREPARATION METHOD: Include in the daily diet (for adults only)
- **Chicory**
  THERAPEUTIC ACTION: Reduces depression, apathy, and exhaustion due to illness or overwork
  PREPARATION METHOD: Standard hot infusion, decoction, fresh plant tincture
- **Cinnamon**
  THERAPEUTIC ACTION: Reduces fatigue, depression, mental dullness, and stress

PREPARATION METHOD: Standard hot infusion, dry plant tincture, herbal wine, herbal bath

- **Cloves**

    THERAPEUTIC ACTION: Reduces weakness and depression

    PREPARATION METHOD: Standard hot infusion, decoction, dry plant tincture, herbal bath

- **Fennel seed**

    THERAPEUTIC ACTION: Acts as a sedative

    PREPARATION METHOD: Standard hot infusion, decoction, dry plant tincture, herbal bath

- **Marjoram**

    THERAPEUTIC ACTION: Reduces emotional tension and anxiety, agitated depression, insomnia, mental weakness, and vertigo

    PREPARATION METHOD: Standard hot infusion, dry plant tincture, herbal wine, herbal bath

- **Nutmeg**

    THERAPEUTIC ACTION: Good for all nervous ailments

    PREPARATION METHOD: Standard hot infusion, decoction, dry plant tincture, herbal bath

- **Rosemary**

    THERAPEUTIC ACTION: Reduces fatigue; strengthens body and mind

    PREPARATION METHOD: Standard hot infusion, decoction, fresh plant tincture, dry plant tincture, herbal bath

- **Sage**

    THERAPEUTIC ACTION: Reduces nervousness and anxiety, vertigo, nervous exhaustion, restlessness, agitated depression, and insomnia (for insomnia, use sage with bruised cloves); aids memory

    PREPARATION METHOD: Standard hot infusion, fresh plant tincture, herbal wine, herbal bath

- **Thyme and rosemary**

    THERAPEUTIC ACTION: Reduces fatigue, depression, and nervous exhaustion

    PREPARATION METHOD: Standard hot infusion, fresh plant tincture, dry plant tincture, herbal bath

Foods

- **Celery**

    THERAPEUTIC ACTION: Reduces fatigue and nervousness; strengthens nerves and adrenal glands

    PREPARATION METHOD: Fresh plant tincture

- **Lemon**

  THERAPEUTIC ACTION: Strengthens nerves

  PREPARATION METHOD: Include in the daily diet

- **Lettuce**

  THERAPEUTIC ACTION: Reduces depression and anxiety

  PREPARATION METHOD: Decoction, fresh plant tincture

- **Oats**

  THERAPEUTIC ACTION: Reduces depression, exhaustion, and anxiety; lifts spirits; increases nerve strength; promotes restfulness

  PREPARATION METHOD: Include in the daily diet

- **Pumpkin seeds**

  THERAPEUTIC ACTION: Reduces depression and insomnia

  PREPARATION METHOD: Fresh plant tincture, dry plant tincture; include in the daily diet

Reflexology

For instructions on reflexology, see "Reflexology" under "How to Use the Therapy Section" at the beginning of Part II.

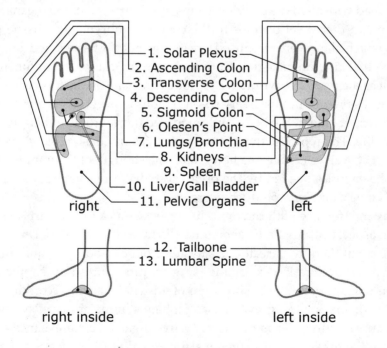

1. Solar Plexus
2. Ascending Colon
3. Transverse Colon
4. Descending Colon
5. Sigmoid Colon
6. Olesen's Point
7. Lungs/Bronchia
8. Kidneys
9. Spleen
10. Liver/Gall Bladder
11. Pelvic Organs
12. Tailbone
13. Lumbar Spine

right   left

right inside   left inside

REPRODUCTIVE HEALTH

TEACHING

Our reproductive organs are the miraculous center of all our biological processes. The Reproductive Organ System forms the most intimate network in the body, and is the hidden partner of all other organ systems. This system is responsible for the primary biological vitality of the body; it serves as the foundation of the immune system and is involved in the basic nutrition of all cells.

Embryological Development of the Reproductive Organs

The complex tissues of the reproductive organs are developed from all three of the original embryological tissues: some from the ectoderm, some from the mesoderm, and some from the endoderm. All of the body's systems develop from these tissue systems, but the fact that the reproductive organs develop from *all three tissue systems* means that they greatly influence the functions associated with all of the body's systems. After birth, all of the organs and tissues retain their relationships to the original embryological tissue system from which they were produced, meaning that all tissues and organs are related first and foremost to their own embryological system of functions.

Just as the reproductive organs reproduce new life in the form of offspring, so they also reproduce us. Every second, thousands of cells in our bodies die and, every moment, the body and mind need to reproduce themselves and renew life. The reproductive system conceives us constantly just as it does when it conceives the life of a new child. The strength of the immune system and the energies needed by the organ systems to regenerate the body and mind come from the reproductive organs.

Any interference with the reproductive system causes disturbances in all major aspects of our body and mind. Birth control pills, IUDs, hormone replacement therapy, vasectomies, hysterectomies, abortions, and the possible scar tissue from D&Cs or other surgical procedures in the reproductive organs damage or inhibit the functions of this vital system. According to Classical medicine, anything that causes problems in major organ systems will also cause disturbances in the reproductive organs. This imbalance happens because the organ systems contain a functional feedback loop to the reproductive organs.

For example, the Large Intestine System controls the basic energies of the pelvic organs in their ability to excrete. The ability to menstruate, have a bowel movement, and urinate, as well as the function of orgasm and giving birth, are all part of the Large Intestine System. Disorders such as chronic low back problems or chronic constipation can inhibit the important functions of the large intestine system, but so can reproductive organ cysts and fibromas. These problems are associated with chronic disturbances of functional energies in the pelvic organs and the basic energies of the central nervous system. Conversely, when signals from the nerve system constantly overstimulate reproductive organ tissues, cysts and fibromas can develop. Stress also affects the nerve system and can build toxins in nerve tissues, causing them to function poorly and contribute to the formation of cysts and fibromas.

Reproductive Organs and Energies

The Stomach/Spleen System creates processes from the digestion and metabolism of food. This energy is stored in the kidneys and produces the sexual vitality of the egg and semen, allowing us to reproduce offspring. The Stomach/Spleen System directly affects the reproductive organs by nourishing them and keeping their functions strong. Current research shows that nonorganic, denatured foods contain toxins from pesticides and chemical fertilizers that can create sterility and hereditary problems in offspring. In addition, the Stomach/Spleen System has a direct connection to the function of the breasts and breast tissues. For this reason, breast tumors need to be treated through the reproductive organs and the Stomach/Spleen System.

The Liver/Gallbladder System is also directly connected to the function of the reproductive organs. A special branch of the energies of the Liver/Gallbladder System controls the uterus, ovaries, and testes. This connection explains why toxins associated with alcohol, tobacco, chemical medicines, mercury fillings, and environmental toxins, all of which are detoxified through the liver, are known to create problems for the embryo and contribute to infertility and impotency.

The final energetic products of the reproductive organs are sent directly to the heart, to be dispersed throughout the body. These energies are the basis for the immune system, the vital energy of the body, and the subtle energies of nutrition for all the body's cells.

During embryological development, the reproductive organs are associated with the Kidney/Bladder System. The kidneys store the energy of reproduction that is vital to the testes and ovaries and are also responsible for the energy patterns we inherit from our parents. These hereditary energies not only function in the embryo, but also serve as the foundation for the basic vital energies of the body throughout one's life.

Menopause: A Natural Process

Menopause is a natural process for all mammals. Therefore, it has no negative symptoms and creates no problems in itself. Menopause, like puberty, is an important part of the way the body and mind mature and develop. Problems such as hot flashes, decrease in bone tissue, and depression or mood swings are not the *fault* of menopause, but indicate that one or more of the organ systems that control the functions of the reproductive system are so compromised that they are not able, or do not have the strength, to integrate these natural changes. If these symptoms arise, it is important to treat the systems that cause them through natural means. Hormone replacement therapy has been popular for many years, but current research has pointed out that there are major health risks with this form of treatment. Remember: the natural hormonal changes that accompany menopause are not the *cause* of symptoms. Thus, hormonal imbalances are symptoms caused by the functional disturbances in the organ systems that control hormone balances.

THERAPY

MENSTRUAL CRAMPS AND PREMENSTRUAL SYNDROME

During menstruation, the outer layer of the uterine mucous membranes sheds some of its cells along with the unfertilized egg. This loosening of cells and mucous membrane also produces some light bleeding. The body uses bleeding as a natural way of cleansing its tissues and revitalizing them. During the menstrual process, cramping may occur, which can be a psychological response to bleeding. Fear of bleeding is layered deep in the psyche and can cause contractions of the tissues involved. Blood not only carries nutrients and vital substances to all the tissues but also carries the energies of our identity and the biological integrity of our body. When we bleed, this deep layer of the psyche can feel threatened. In our culture, we associate bleeding with something that is negative, an acute problem the body is having that needs to be quickly resolved. Menstrual bleeding, however, is a natural and healthy process. Many young girls just entering puberty and experiencing their first menstruation are not prepared psychologically to integrate the bleeding process. Therefore, they react unconsciously against this process, resulting in tension and cramping in the tissues of the uterus. If not addressed, this unconscious psychological reaction can persist throughout their lives.

Structural issues can also contribute to cramps. The nerves that cause the uterus to contract and expel the menstrual fluids come from the lower spine. Chronic tension in the lower back or misaligned vertebrae can compromise the nerve signals to the uterus and cause cramping.

All of the major organ systems are connected in a feedback loop to the reproductive organs: Liver/Gallbladder, Kidney/Bladder, Stomach/Spleen/Pancreas, Lung/Colon, and Heart/Small Intestines. Chronic health issues in any of these systems will affect the reproductive organs and may cause menstrual problems, including cramping. In addition, health issues of the uterus and ovaries, such as cysts or fibromas, will also affect the menstrual process. See your natural healthcare professional for advice on these issues.

General Remedies

Remedy #1
- 2 ounces (1 shot glass) aloe vera gel or juice
- $\frac{1}{8}$ teaspoon black pepper

Mix the aloe vera gel or juice with the black pepper. Drink 3 times per day until cramping is better.

Tissue Salts

- *Ferrum phos.* 6X (for pain, vomiting)
- *Kali phos.* 6X (for depression, irritability, nervousness, cramping)
- *Mag. phos.* 6X (for cramping)
- *Natrum mur.* 6X (for pain in the abdomen, headache, vomiting, depression)
- *Silicea* 6X (for backache)
- *Calc. fluor.* 6X (for bearing-down pain, lower abdominal pain)
- *Calc. sulph.* 6X (for headache, weakness)

One or more remedies can be selected from this list depending on your symptoms. Remedies can be taken together if more than one remedy is selected. Take remedies 3–5 times per day; reduce the number of doses as symptoms begin to improve.

Spices, Herbs, and Foods

- **Anise seed**

PREPARATION METHOD: Standard hot infusion, decoction, dry plant tincture, herbal bath

- **Basil**

  PREPARATION METHOD: Standard hot infusion, decoction, fresh plant tincture, dry plant tincture, herbal bath
- **Celery**

  PREPARATION METHOD: Decoction
- **Cinnamon**

  PREPARATION METHOD: Standard hot infusion, decoction, fresh plant tincture, dry plant tincture, herbal bath
- **Fennel seed**

  PREPARATION METHOD: Standard hot infusion, decoction, herbal compress, dry plant tincture, herbal bath
- **Ginger**

  PREPARATION METHOD: Standard hot infusion, decoction, herbal compress, fresh plant tincture, dry plant tincture
- **Oats**

  PREPARATION METHOD: Include in the daily diet
- **Sage**

  PREPARATION METHOD: Standard hot infusion, decoction, herbal compress, fresh plant tincture, dry plant tincture, herbal bath

YEAST INFECTIONS

Yeasts and fungi belong to a group of microbes called mycobacteria, which are part of the metabolic or "digestive" process of all tissue groups. All tissue systems, including the reproductive system, have their own digestive metabolism that nourishes their cells and maintains their health. If the cells of the tissues that are responsible for digesting nutrients are compromised, they will become unhealthy. These unhealthy cells are destroyed and cleaned up by mycobacteria so that the tissues can maintain their vital and healthy cells.

In nature, we see for example, fungi appearing on dead or dying trees. The fungi help nature to clean itself and to support the metabolic processes of the surrounding healthy new growth. The body works the same way. Mycobacteria do not cause disease but are part of nature's way of dealing with diseased or weakened cells and tissues. So-called fungal infections are not really diseases—rather, their symptoms show that a specific tissue is being chronically compromised and cannot maintain its level of health.

Any factor, such as the use of birth control pills, IUDs, or operations in the reproductive organs, as well as functional problems in the organ systems that control the reproductive organs, will compromise the system and tend to produce mycobacteria. As with all other bodily symptoms, it is vital that the causes and not just the symptoms be dealt with properly. Using antifungal medicines, for example, only suppresses the symptoms and compromises the natural way that the body deals with its health issues. These medicines do not cure the cause or contribute to the health of the body, but mask the real reasons for the symptoms. When in doublt about the cause of symptoms, contact your natural healthcare professional.

Tissue Salts

Itching Discharge:

- *Silicea 6X*
- *Natrum mur. 6X*

Take 4–5 times daily for up to three days. Reduce the number of doses as symptoms begin to improve.

Creamy Discharge:

- *Natrum phos. 6X*
- *Calc. phos. 6X*

Take 4–5 times daily for up to three days. Reduce the number of doses as symptoms begin to improve.

Egg-White Discharge:

- *Calc. phos. 6X*

Take 4–5 times daily for up to three days. Reduce the number of doses as symptoms begin to improve.

Milky or Whitish Discharge:

- *Kali mur. 6X*

Take 4–5 times daily for up to three days. Reduce the number of doses as symptoms begin to improve.

Greenish Discharge:

- *Kali sulph. 6X*

Take 4–5 times daily for up to three days. Reduce the number of doses as symptoms begin to improve.

Honey-Colored Discharge:

- *Natrum phos. 6X*

Take 4–5 times daily for up to three days. Reduce the number of doses as symptoms begin to improve.

Yellow Discharge:

- *Kali sulph. 6X*
- *Kali phos. 6X*

Take 4–5 times daily for up to three days. Reduce the number of doses as symptoms begin to improve.

Itching of the Vulva:

* *Natrum mur.* 6X
* *Silicea* 6X

Take 4–5 times daily for up to three days. Reduce the number of doses as symptoms begin to improve.

Spices, Herbs, and Foods

* **Cinnamon**

  PREPARATION METHOD: Standard hot infusion, decoction, fresh plant tincture, dry plant tincture, herbal bath

* **Fennel seed**

  PREPARATION METHOD: Standard hot infusion, decoction, herbal compress, dry plant tincture, herbal bath

* **Garlic**

  PREPARATION METHOD: Garlic oil

* **Ginger**

  PREPARATION METHOD: Standard hot infusion, decoction, herbal compress, fresh plant tincture, dry plant tincture

* **Honey**

  PREPARATION METHOD: Use as ointment for sores at the opening of the vagina

* **Parsley**

  PREPARATION METHOD: Standard hot infusion, decoction, fresh plant tincture, dry plant tincture, herbal bath

* **Sage**

  PREPARATION METHOD: Standard hot infusion, decoction, herbal compress, fresh plant tincture, dry plant tincture, herbal bath

* **Thyme**

  PREPARATION METHOD: Standard hot infusion, decoction, fresh plant tincture, dry plant tincture, herbal bath

GENITAL HERPES

See "Herpes" on page 246.

INFERTILITY AND IMPOTENCY

Infertility and impotency are not usually problems that originate in the reproductive organs themselves. The exceptions are dysfunctional tissues with problems such as cysts, fibromas, or tumors. More often, impotency and infertility are caused by chronic disturbances and health issues in the organ systems. All five major organ systems share vital functions with the reproductive organs. Chronic gastric issues, lung and breathing problems, chronic stress, and toxic loads (including medical drugs) on tissues can all cause impotency and infertility. When attempting to resolve chronic health problems, the body uses its vital energies to heal itself and regenerate its systems. The energies it usually uses for menstruation and sexual activity are then redirected to the more vital process of healing.

Frequently, people with chronic mental or physical health issues will take drugs to deal with the problems. Even though the symptoms might be alleviated by drugs, chemical drugs will not cure the issue and will have side effects. The body then has to continually work on healing the original issues plus deal with the side effects of the drugs. This will severely limit the reproductive energies that are necessary for potency and fertility. See your natural healthcare professional to address issues of this nature.

Tissue Salts

Painful Menses in Connection with Infertility:
- *Calc. phos. 6X*
- *Kali phos. 6X*
- *Mag. phos. 6X*
- *Ferrum phos. 6X*
- *Natrum mur. 6X*

Take 3–4 times daily for up to three days. Reduce the number of doses as symptoms begin to improve.

Sterility:
- *Silicea 6X*
- *Natrum phos. 6X*

Take twice daily for up to three weeks.

Impotency:
- *Kali phos. 6X*
- *Natrum mur. 6X*

Take twice daily for up to three weeks.

Spice and Herbs

- **Basil**

  PREPARATION METHOD: Standard hot infusion, decoction, fresh plant tincture, dry plant tincture, herbal bath

- **Black pepper**
  PREPARATION METHOD: Include in the daily diet
- **Celery seed**
  PREPARATION METHOD: Decoction
- **Cinnamon**
  PREPARATION METHOD: Standard hot infusion, decoction, fresh plant tincture, dry plant tincture, herbal bath
- **Cloves**
  PREPARATION METHOD: Standard hot infusion, dry plant tincture, herbal wine, herbal bath
- **Marjoram**
  PREPARATION METHOD: Standard hot infusion, decoction, dry plant tincture, herbal wine, herbal bath
- **Rosemary**
  PREPARATION METHOD: Standard hot infusion, decoction, fresh plant tincture, dry plant tincture, herbal bath
- **Thyme**
  PREPARATION METHOD: Standard hot infusion, decoction, fresh plant tincture, dry plant tincture, herbal bath

Foods

- **Asparagus**
  PREPARATION METHOD: Include in the daily diet
- **Oats**
  PREPARATION METHOD: Include in the daily diet

GENERAL CARE OF THE REPRODUCTIVE SYSTEM

Spices and Herbs

- **Anise seed**
  THERAPEUTIC ACTION: Relieves painful menstruation and cramps
  PREPARATION METHOD: Standard hot infusion, decoction, dry plant tincture, herbal bath
- **Basil**
  THERAPEUTIC ACTION: Relieves painful menstruation and cramps; promotes menses, libido, and fertility; reduces impotency
  PREPARATION METHOD: Standard hot infusion, decoction, fresh plant tincture, dry plant tincture, herbal bath

- **Black pepper**

  THERAPEUTIC ACTION: Reduces impotency; helps relieve prolapsed uterus

  PREPARATION METHOD: Include in the daily diet

- **Celery seed**

  THERAPEUTIC ACTION: Relieves painful menstruation and cramps; restores the uterus; promotes menses; stimulates potency and fertility

  PREPARATION METHOD: Decoction

- **Cinnamon**

  THERAPEUTIC ACTION: Relieves frigidity and impotence, painful menstruation, and cramps; antifungal and anti-*Candida*

  PREPARATION METHOD: Standard hot infusion, decoction, herbal compress, herbal oil, herbal bath

- **Cloves**

  THERAPEUTIC ACTION: Increases libido

  PREPARATION METHOD: Standard hot infusion, dry plant tincture, herbal wine, herbal bath

- **Fennel seed**

  THERAPEUTIC ACTION: Stimulates the uterus; promotes menses; relieves painful menstruation and cramps; reduces estrogen insufficiency; antifungal and anti-*Candida*

  PREPARATION METHOD: Standard hot infusion, decoction, herbal compress, dry plant tincture, herbal bath

- **Garlic**

  THERAPEUTIC ACTION: Antifungal

  PREPARATION METHOD: Garlic oil

- **Ginger**

  THERAPEUTIC ACTION: Relieves painful menstruation and cramps; supports the uterus; relieves *Trichomonas* infections

  PREPARATION METHOD: Standard hot infusion, decoction, herbal compress, fresh plant tincture, dry plant tincture

- **Marjoram**

  THERAPEUTIC ACTION: Lowers excessive libido; stimulates fertility; relieves painful menstruation

  PREPARATION METHOD: Standard hot infusion, decoction, dry plant tincture, herbal wine, herbal bath

- **Parsley**

  THERAPEUTIC ACTION: Antifungal; uterine tonic

  PREPARATION METHOD: Standard hot infusion, decoction, fresh plant tincture, dry plant tincture, herbal bath

- **Rosemary**

  THERAPEUTIC ACTION: Reproductive organ tonic

  PREPARATION METHOD: Standard hot infusion, decoction, fresh plant tincture, dry plant tincture, herbal bath

- **Sage**

  THERAPEUTIC ACTION: Relieves painful menses and menopause problems; helps restore estrogen; antifungal; relieves genital herpes

  PREPARATION METHOD: Standard hot infusion, decoction, herbal compress, fresh plant tincture, dry plant tincture, herbal bath

- **Savory**

  THERAPEUTIC ACTION: Antifungal

  PREPARATION METHOD: Decoction, herbal compress, herbal oil, herbal bath

- **Thyme**

  THERAPEUTIC ACTION: Stimulates the uterus; promotes menses; increases libido; relieves fungal infections

  PREPARATION METHOD: Standard hot infusion, decoction, fresh plant tincture, dry plant tincture, herbal bath

Foods

- **Asparagus**

  THERAPEUTIC ACTION: Relieves vaginal dryness; enhances libido; reduces impotency

  PREPARATION METHOD: Include in the daily diet

- **Honey**

  THERAPEUTIC ACTION: Antimicrobial; stimulates the healing process in skin and membranes

  PREPARATION METHOD: Use as an ointment for sores at opening of the vagina

- **Oats**

  THERAPEUTIC ACTION: Strengthens the reproductive system; relieves menstrual cramps; reduces estrogen insufficiency

  PREPARATION METHOD: Include in the daily diet

- **Estrogenic enhancers:** Anise, apple, broccoli, brussels sprouts, cabbage, cauliflower, corn, cumin, flaxseed, garlic, licorice, oats, peanuts, pineapple, potatoes, rice, and sesame seed

Reflexology

For instructions on reflexology, see "Reflexology" under "How to Use the Therapy Section" at the beginning of Part II.

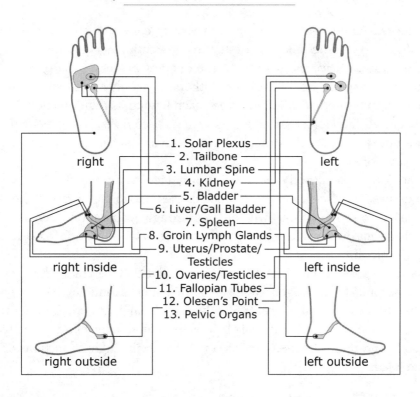

1. Solar Plexus
2. Tailbone
3. Lumbar Spine
4. Kidney
5. Bladder
6. Liver/Gall Bladder
7. Spleen
8. Groin Lymph Glands
9. Uterus/Prostate/Testicles
10. Ovaries/Testicles
11. Fallopian Tubes
12. Olesen's Point
13. Pelvic Organs

right

left

right inside

left inside

right outside

left outside

SKIN PROBLEMS

TEACHING

We tend to consider the skin as nothing more than a covering for the body that is a container for an assortment of important organs and tissues. Actually, the skin is the *largest* organ of the body and plays a major role in the functioning of both the body and mind.

The skin is developed in the embryo from the ectoderm, the same embryological tissue from which the brain, nerves, hair, and nails develop. It is through the tissues of the ectoderm that the body becomes sensitive to the world that surrounds us and in which we move. Through the skin, nerve tissues, and sensory stimulation, we not only respond to signals coming from all our tissue systems, but we truly touch the world.

The connection between the brain, nerve system, and the skin becomes apparent when we blush or turn pale. The skin acts as a defusing mechanism for the central nervous system by transferring compromising factors away from the nerve tissues and into itself, thus preventing nerve damage.

The skin participates in some of the deepest processes that govern the health and maintenance of the body. Although we only see the surface of the skin, it is composed of different layers, each having its own function. It contains growth and pigment layers as well as a complex nerve system that forms our sense of touch. Moreover, it has a layer that contains the blood and lymph vessels.

The skin helps the body maintain a normal temperature in its inner organs and tissues. The circulation of our blood carries heat to the surface of the skin, where it is cooled by contact with air and through evaporation. Such transference happens during a fever, when heat moves to the skin surface in order to cool the blood.

When exposed to sunlight, the skin reacts and changes color. This tanning process results from an agent called melanin, which is found in the skin's connective tissues. Melanin is controlled by the pineal gland, a very important gland in the midbrain. The pineal gland helps maintain the harmony between all body and mind functions and is connected to the higher functions of the mind itself.

Skin: The Classical Medicine Viewpoint

In Ayurveda, the skin is called "the organ that digests." This phrase relates to the fact that the skin absorbs everything with which it comes into contact. Many natural therapies include rubbing substances into the skin or bathing the limbs or entire body. The purpose of such therapy is not so much to help the skin, but to use the skin as a vehicle to transfer therapeutic substances to the organs via the blood and nerve systems. On the other hand, the skin's ability to absorb means that the toxins found in lotions, sunscreens, perfumes, and deodorants are carried directly into our bloodstream and damage our sensitive cells and tissues.

The dynamic energy of the lungs and the metabolic process of breathing directly affect the skin's ability to adapt to varying external conditions such as cold, heat, dampness, and dryness. If the lung system is not functioning properly, we can develop colds, flu, and disorders connected with sweating. Proper breathing can maintain lung functions and support the work of the skin.

The Stomach/Spleen System also has a strong effect on the skin. This system involves digesting and transporting fluid nutrients throughout the body.

If the Stomach/Spleen System is compromised, the skin will not receive the energy and nutrients it needs and will function poorly. Eating properly and taking care of our digestion enables the processes in the skin to perform well and maintain health.

The skin, through the functions of the heart and circulatory system, reflects the health of the entire organism. In Chinese medicine, the heart is called "the root of life." The heart controls the blood vessels, which carry the essence of all the life-building processes of the body. When the heart system is compromised, this is reflected in the skin as an unhealthy pallor. We often intuitively perceive this imbalance when we see someone who looks pale.

The Liver/Gallbladder System also influences the functions of the skin. The liver controls the vital health of the skin as a whole. Whenever the liver is burdened by toxins or is not functioning well, the skin will lose its luster, become dry and brittle, or develop eczema from the burden of toxins in the Liver System. Maintaining the health of the liver is essential for the health of the skin.

THERAPY

SUN PROTECTION

Sunlight nourishes the whole body as well as the skin. When we've been inside all winter, for instance, our skin becomes pale and lacks the luster and life it has when we are able to be out in the sun. Too much sun, however, can harm the skin with excess drying and heating energies. It is always a good idea to stay in shade as much as possible, and wear light, loose-fitting clothes when in climates that have strong, hot sunlight.

Oils are very good for the skin. After having been in the sun, rub a mixture of almond and olive oils onto the skin. This will restore the skin and keep it healthy. Avoid sunscreens and sun lotions—they contain toxins and do not contribute to the health of the skin.

General Remedies

Remedy for Skin Rejuvenation after Sun Exposure:
- 1 part almond oil
- 1 part olive oil

Mix the almond oil with the olive oil. Apply to the skin. Allow the skin to absorb the oil for 15 minutes to reduce heat and enliven skin tissues, then wipe away any excess.

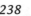

Remedy for Skin Rejuvenation during Winter:
- Sesame oil

Apply oil to skin. Allow the skin to absorb the oil for 15 minutes, then wipe away any excess. This oil builds up all seven layers of the skin tissues and restores their functions.

BOILS

Boils are inflammations of the hair follicles, which are part of the skin's deeper tissue system. They can occur when the skin is not properly cleaned or when using substances that contain toxins and clog the skin, such as makeup, lotions, or deodorants. As with other cases, in which microbes are involved, the microbe itself is not the cause; rather it is a response to the damage being done to tissues and cells. The microbes respond to whatever factor is compromising the tissue; this creates a strong immune reaction that brings lymphatic fluids and white blood cells to the area, producing swelling and pus.

The following suggestions will help resolve the boil. It is important to note, however, that skin can be *too* clean! Using antibiotic soaps or lotions, or washing the skin too often with soaps or cleansers, will remove the natural oils and substances that protect and nourish the skin.

General Remedies

Remedy #1
- 1 teaspoon onion, cooked
- ⅛ teaspoon ginger powder
- ⅛ teaspoon turmeric (if available)
- 1 teaspoon olive oil

To bring a skin boil to a head, mix the cooked onion, ginger powder, and turmeric (if you have it) with the olive oil and apply directly to the boil.

Remedy #2
- 1 teaspoon wheat flour
- ⅛ teaspoon salt

Mix enough water with the wheat flour to make a paste. Add the salt. Apply to the boil.

Tissue Salts
- *Mag. phos.* 6X
- *Silicea* 6X
- *Ferrum phos.* 6X

- *Kali mur.* 6X

Take these remedies together 4–5 times a day for two to three days. Reduce the number of doses as symptoms begin to improve.

Spices and Herbs

- **Basil**
  PREPARATION METHOD: Herbal compress
- **Cayenne pepper**
  PREPARATION METHOD: Include in the daily diet
- **Cinnamon**
  PREPARATION METHOD: Herbal compress
- **Garlic**
  PREPARATION METHOD: Garlic oil
- **Sage**
  PREPARATION METHOD: Herbal compress, herbal bath
- **Savory**
  PREPARATION METHOD: Herbal compress, fresh plant tincture, dry plant tincture, herbal bath
- **Thyme**
  PREPARATION METHOD: Herbal compress, fresh plant tincture, dry plant tincture, herbal oil, herbal bath

Foods

- **Carrots**
  PREPARATION METHOD: Vegetable compress
- **Cashew nuts**
  PREPARATION METHOD: Make a compress by crushing cashew nuts and placing in a bowl. Pour enough boiling water over to just cover them. Steep for 10 minutes. Place directly on the boil and hold in place with a cloth.
- **Flaxseed**
  PREPARATION METHOD: To bring a boil to a head, crush whole flaxseeds and mix into a paste with butter. Apply to site; replace daily.
- **Lettuce**
  PREPARATION METHOD: Vegetable compress (to prepare compress, boil lettuce in olive oil for 10 minutes; strain, and place directly on site)
- **Oats**
  PREPARATION METHOD: Boil two quarts of water with two cups of oatmeal. Simmer for 15 minutes in a covered pan; strain liquid. Pour liquid into bath or let cool and use as a wash on the skin, as needed.

- **Onion**

  PREPARATION METHOD: Vegetable compress

- **Pineapple**

  PREPARATION METHOD: Fruit compress

ECZEMA AND FUNGAL INFECTIONS

All healing processes work from the inside out and the skin plays an important role in these. Rashes, eruptions on the skin, and eczema are not skin "diseases" but a symptom of the body healing itself from internal factors that are compromising organs and tissues. As the body heals, it cleanses, moving toxins from the inner tissues to the outside tissues—the skin.

The skin is connected to the ectoderm embryological tissue that produces the nerve system and the large intestine controls the basic energies of the nerve system. Just as the large intestine gathers waste products and toxins left from the digestive process and eliminates them to the outside through bowel movements, so the skin gathers and pushes toxins from the inner tissues to the outside, causing symptoms like rashes and eczema while the cleansing occurs.

Chronic eczema shows that the body is producing or is continually exposed to toxins, such as the toxins from mercury fillings, or that one or more of the organ systems is not functioning properly and is generating toxins from incomplete metabolic processes. Often things that come into direct contact with the body, like rings, jewelry, and watchbands, can react with the skin and produce contact symptoms.

Fungal infections on the skin are due to the presence of mycobacteria. The fungus is not the *cause* of the problem, but a healing *response* to factors that are damaging the metabolic cells and tissues of the skin. We can see this clearly in nature. Wherever there is fungus, on trees or plants for example, we observe that the trees or plants are dying. When organic organisms can no longer digest and metabolize well, they will die. Fungus microbes clean up dead and dying tissues in our environment as well as in our bodies. This microbial response is usually caused by toxins that cause damage to the body's ability to digest and transform nutrients. These toxins can be from drugs, nonorganic foods, the environment, and the toxins that occur from incomplete processes due to functional disturbances of the organ systems. It is important not to suppress skin symptoms (through topical drugs, for example) as that will drive the reaction and the toxins back into the vital tissues, inhibiting the natural healing process. Natural topical remedies can be used to support this process and relieve the symptoms without interfering with healing.

General Remedies

Remedy #1

- 1 teaspoon ground coriander
- 1 cup boiling water

Steep the ground coriander in boiling water. Drink 2 cups per day for up to a week.

Remedy #2

- 1 tablespoon cornstarch
- Rose water (if available)

Mix the cornstarch with enough rose water (if you have it) or plain water to make a paste. This can be applied 1–3 times daily. Do not cover.

Tissue Salts

For Eczema:

- *Natrum mur. 6X*
- *Silicea 6X*
- *Natrum phos. 6X*
- *Kali phos. 6X*

Take these remedies together 3 times per day for up to three weeks. Reduce the number of doses as symptoms begin to improve.

For Fungus:

- *Natrum mur. 6X*
- *Kali mur. 6X*

Taken these remedies together 3 times per day for up to three weeks. Reduce the number of doses as symptoms begin to improve.

Spices and Herbs

- **Basil**
  PREPARATION METHOD: Herbal compress
- **Caraway**
  PREPARATION METHOD: Herbal compress, herbal oil, herbal bath
- **Cayenne pepper**
  PREPARATION METHOD: Include in the daily diet
- **Chicory**
  PREPARATION METHOD: Herbal compress, dry plant tincture, herbal bath

- **Cinnamon**
PREPARATION METHOD: Herbal compress
- **Garlic**
PREPARATION METHOD: Garlic oil
- **Oregano**
PREPARATION METHOD: Herbal compress, fresh plant tincture, dry plant tincture, herbal oil, herbal bath
- **Parsley**
PREPARATION METHOD: Herbal compress
- **Savory**
PREPARATION METHOD: Herbal compress, fresh plant tincture, dry plant tincture, herbal bath
- **Thyme**
PREPARATION METHOD: Herbal compress, fresh plant tincture, dry plant tincture, herbal oil, herbal bath
- **Turmeric**
PREPARATION METHOD: Herbal compress, herbal oil

Foods

- **Avocado**
PREPARATION METHOD: Mash fresh avocado; place directly on the site and hold in place with a cloth.
- **Beets**
PREPARATION METHOD: Vegetable compress
- **Buckwheat**
PREPARATION METHOD: Add enough hot water to buckwheat flour to make a mushy paste. Cover the site with the paste and hold in place with a cloth.
- **Cabbage**
PREPARATION METHOD: Vegetable compress
- **Carrots**
PREPARATION METHOD: Vegetable compress
- **Cashew nuts**
PREPARATION METHOD: Make a compress by crushing cashew nuts and placing in a bowl. Pour enough boiling water into the bowl to just cover the nuts. Steep 10 minutes. Place directly on the site and hold in place with a cloth.
- **Celery**
PREPARATION METHOD: Vegetable compress
- **Lemon**
PREPARATION METHOD: Fruit juice application

- **Oats**

PREPARATION METHOD: Boil 2 quarts of water with 2 cups of oatmeal. Simmer for 15 minutes in a covered pan; strain liquid. Pour the liquid into a bath or let it cool and use as wash on the skin, as needed.

- **Turnips**

PREPARATION METHOD: Vegetable compress

RASH

Skin rashes are not skin diseases but inflammations that indicate the skin is reacting to contact with an irritant or toxin. Rashes also can occur when the body cleanses toxins from its tissues by way of the skin. In addition, a rash may occur as part of the healing reaction in so-called childhood diseases. Rashes should never be suppressed but allowed to resolve naturally.

Tissue Salts

- *Natrum phos.* 6X
- *Ferrum phos.* 6X
- *Kali sulph.* 6X
- *Silicea* 6X

Take these remedies together 3 times a day for up to a week. Reduce the number of doses as symptoms begin to improve.

Spices, Herbs, and Foods

- **Avocado**

PREPARATION METHOD: Mash fresh avocado; place directly on the site and hold in place with a cloth.

- **Buckwheat**

PREPARATION METHOD: Add enough hot water to buckwheat flour to make a mushy paste. Cover the site with the paste and hold in place with a cloth.

- **Cabbage**

PREPARATION METHOD: Vegetable compress

- **Cucumber**

PREPARATION METHOD: Cut slices of fresh cucumber; place directly on the skin and hold in place with a cloth.

- **Lemon**

PREPARATION METHOD: Fruit juice application

- **Oats**

PREPARATION METHOD: Boil 2 quarts of water with 2 cups of oatmeal. Simmer for 15 minutes in a covered pan; strain liquid. Pour the liquid into a bath or let it cool and use as wash on the skin, as needed.

- **Potato**

  PREPARATION METHOD: Cut thin slices of raw potato; place directly on the site and hold in place with a cloth.

HIVES

Hives are not a skin disease but an immune reaction in the connective tissues of the skin layers. The immune system produces fluids that contain immune substances and nutrients for all layers of the skin. When skin and connective cells are compromised, the immune system increases this fluid around the cells, producing local swelling. Hives can also appear as an allergic reaction to toxins or from exposure to climatic factors like cold. If you experience hives when in contact with a nontoxic natural substance, it indicates that there is a chronic problem in your immune system and you need to address this issue by contacting a natural healthcare professional.

Tissue Salts

- *Natrum phos.* 6X
- *Natrum sulph.* 6X
- *Ferrum phos.* 6X
- *Kali phos.* 6X

  Take these remedies together 4–5 times per day for up to two days. Reduce the number of doses as symptoms begin to improve.

Spices and Herbs

- **Ginger**

  PREPARATION METHOD: Herbal compress, herbal bath

PSORIASIS

Psoriasis is a true skin disease. Its patterns lie dormant in the deeper constitutional levels of the organism and are activated by factors such as vaccines, medical drugs, mercury fillings, environmental toxins, and toxins from nonorganic foods, which compromise the immune system and organ functions. To deal with the causes of psoriasis, see a natural healthcare professional and use the suggestions below.

Tissue Salts

For Itching:

- *Calc. phos.* 6X
- *Kali sulph.* 6X
- *Kali phos.* 6X
- *Silicea* 6X

Take these remedies together 3 times per day for up to two weeks. Reduce the number of doses as symptoms begin to improve.

Spices and Herbs

- **Parsley**

  PREPARATION METHOD: Herbal compress

- **Turmeric**

  PREPARATION METHOD: Herbal compress, herbal oil

Foods

- **Avocado**

  PREPARATION METHOD: Mash fresh avocado; place directly on the site and hold in place with a cloth.

- **Beets**

  PREPARATION METHOD: Vegetable compress

- **Buckwheat**

  PREPARATION METHOD: Add enough hot water to buckwheat flour to make a mushy paste. Cover the site with the paste and hold in place with a cloth.

- **Cashew nuts**

  PREPARATION METHOD: Make a compress by crushing cashew nuts and placing in bowl. Pour enough boiling water to just cover them. Steep 10 minutes. Place directly on the site and hold in place with a cloth.

- **Cucumber**

  PREPARATION METHOD: Cut slices of fresh cucumber; place directly on the skin and hold in place with a cloth.

- **Oats**

  PREPARATION METHOD: Boil 2 quarts of water with 2 cups of oatmeal. Simmer for 15 minutes in a covered pan; strain the liquid. Pour the liquid into a bath or let it cool and use as wash on the skin, as needed.

- **Olive oil**

  PREPARATION METHOD: Rub skin with olive oil

HERPES

Herpes symptoms can appear in a number of different tissues, such as the skin, eyes, nose, and reproductive organs. Herpes is not a skin disease—it is a viral reaction taking place as part of an immune response. Viruses are always connected to acute or chronic disturbances in the nerve system. This is why herpes outbreaks are often connected to periods of stress. When there are strong stresses on the brain and nerve systems, the immune system reacts through the herpes virus and transfers the stress on the nerve tissues to the skin as part of the healing process. Remember that the skin and nerve tissues were created from the same embryological tissue, the ectoderm, and are therefore connected in their functions.

Tissue Salts

- *Calc. phos.* 6X
- *Calc. sulph.* 6X
- *Natrum mur.* 6X

Take these remedies together 3–8 times per day for up to three weeks. Reduce the number of doses as symptoms begin to improve.

Spices, Herbs, and Foods

- **Garlic**
  PREPARATION METHOD: Garlic oil
- **Oats**
  PREPARATION METHOD: Boil 2 quarts of water with 2 cups of oatmeal. Simmer for 15 minutes in a covered pan; strain liquid. Pour the liquid into a bath or let it cool and use as wash on the skin, as needed.
- **Sage**
  PREPARATION METHOD: Herbal compress, herbal bath

GENERAL CARE OF THE SKIN

Spices and Herbs

- **Basil**
  THERAPEUTIC ACTION: Skin antiseptic; toner; cleanser; enhances healing mechanisms; good for slow-healing wounds
  PREPARATION METHOD: Herbal compress
- **Caraway**
  THERAPEUTIC ACTION: Relieves parasitic skin conditions

PREPARATION METHOD: Herbal compress, herbal oil, herbal bath

- **Cayenne pepper**
  THERAPEUTIC ACTION: Promotes healing of psoriasis and suppurating wounds
  PREPARATION METHOD: Include in the daily diet
- **Chicory**
  THERAPEUTIC ACTION: Relieves skin eruptions
  PREPARATION METHOD: Herbal compress, dry plant tincture, herbal bath
- **Cinnamon**
  THERAPEUTIC ACTION: Relieves *Staphylococcus* infections; antibiotic
  PREPARATION METHOD: Herbal compress
- **Clove and rosemary**
  THERAPEUTIC ACTION: Relieves scabies
  PREPARATION METHOD: Herbal compress, herbal bath
- **Fennel seeds**
  THERAPEUTIC ACTION: Relieves skin fungus
  PREPARATION METHOD: Herbal compress, herbal bath
- **Garlic**
  THERAPEUTIC ACTION: Relieves tinea capitus, ringworm, wounds, abscesses, skin ulcers, gangrene, and varicose veins; stimulates circulation; treats genital warts
  PREPARATION METHOD: Garlic oil (For warts, cut a small sliver of fresh garlic and place on the wart; hold in place with a bandage and replace once a day as necessary.)
- **Ginger**
  THERAPEUTIC ACTION: Reduces hives
  PREPARATION METHOD: Herbal compress, herbal bath
- **Oregano**
  THERAPEUTIC ACTION: Soothes itchy skin; relieves parasitic skin diseases, sores, and skin ulcers
  PREPARATION METHOD: Herbal compress, fresh plant tincture, dry plant tincture, herbal oil, herbal bath
- **Parsley**
  THERAPEUTIC ACTION: Relieves psoriasis
  PREPARATION METHOD: Herbal compress
- **Rosemary**
  THERAPEUTIC ACTION: External skin stimulant; use as a hair conditioner and body wash
  PREPARATION METHOD: Decoction, herbal bath

- **Sage**
  THERAPEUTIC ACTION: Relieves chronic skin ulcers, skin sores, abscesses, herpes, and varicose veins
  PREPARATION METHOD: Herbal compress, herbal bath
- **Savory**
  THERAPEUTIC ACTION: Antifungal; antibacterial
  PREPARATION METHOD: Herbal compress, fresh plant tincture, dry plant tincture, herbal bath
- **Thyme**
  THERAPEUTIC ACTION: Helps resolve acne, dermatitis, boils, and abscesses
  PREPARATION METHOD: Herbal compress, fresh plant tincture, dry plant tincture, herbal oil, herbal bath
- **Turmeric**
  THERAPEUTIC ACTION: Relieves itching skin
  PREPARATION METHOD: Herbal compress, herbal oil

Foods

- **Apple cider vinegar** (preferably organic)
  THERAPEUTIC ACTION: Relieves athlete's foot
  PREPARATION METHOD: Soak feet in vinegar once daily
- **Avocado**
  THERAPEUTIC ACTION: Relieves eczema, itching, and dry skin
  PREPARATION METHOD: Mash fresh avocado; place directly on the site and hold in place with a cloth.
- **Beets**
  THERAPEUTIC ACTION: Adjusts pH (acidity) of the skin
  PREPARATION METHOD: Vegetable compress
- **Buckwheat**
  THERAPEUTIC ACTION: Relieves itching rash
  PREPARATION METHOD: Add enough hot water to buckwheat flour to make a mushy paste. Cover the site with the paste and hold in place with a cloth.
- **Cabbage**
  THERAPEUTIC ACTION: Reduces acne and skin inflammation
  PREPARATION METHOD: Vegetable compress
- **Carrots**
  THERAPEUTIC ACTION: Relieves eczema and abscesses
  PREPARATION METHOD: Vegetable compress
- **Cashew nuts**
  THERAPEUTIC ACTION: Relieves ulcers, cracking skin, vesicular eruptions

PREPARATION METHOD: Make a compress by crushing cashew nuts and placing in bowl. Pour enough boiling water to just cover them. Steep 10 minutes. Place directly on the site and hold in place with a cloth.

- **Celery**

  THERAPEUTIC ACTION: Relieves rashes

  PREPARATION METHOD: Vegetable compress

- **Cucumber**

  THERAPEUTIC ACTION: Stimulates and restores healthy skin function

  PREPARATION METHOD: Cut slices of fresh cucumber; place directly on the skin and hold in place with a cloth.

- **Flaxseed and butter**

  THERAPEUTIC ACTION: Stimulates and restores healthy skin function

  PREPARATION METHOD: To bring a boil to a head, crush whole flaxseeds and mix into a paste with butter. Apply to site; replace daily.

- **Lemon**

  THERAPEUTIC ACTION: Relieves ringworm and seborrhea; strengthens skin; relieves rashes and sunburn; reduces blackheads

  PREPARATION METHOD: Fruit juice application

- **Lettuce**

  THERAPEUTIC ACTION: Relieves acne, boils, and abscesses

  PREPARATION METHOD: Vegetable compress (To prepare compress, place lettuce in a pan and cover with olive oil. Simmer for 10 minutes; strain. When comfortably warm, place lettuce directly on the site.)

- **Oats**

  THERAPEUTIC ACTION: Relieves dermatitis, shingles/herpes, eczema, sores, skin inflammation, and skin itch; restores healthy function of the skin

  PREPARATION METHOD: Boil 2 quarts of water with 2 cups of oatmeal. Simmer for 15 minutes in a covered pan; strain liquid. Pour the liquid into a bath or let it cool and use as wash on the skin, as needed.

- **Olive oil**

  THERAPEUTIC ACTION: Protects and rejuvenates skin

  PREPARATION METHOD: Rub skin with olive oil

- **Onion**

  THERAPEUTIC ACTION: Reduces warts; antiseptic for wounds

  PREPARATION METHOD: Vegetable compress

- **Pineapple**

  THERAPEUTIC ACTION: Relieves ulcers; enhances immune process in slow-healing wounds

  PREPARATION METHOD: Fruit compress

- **Potato**
  THERAPEUTIC ACTION: Relieves skin inflammation
  PREPARATION METHOD: Cut thin slices of raw potato; place directly on the site
- **Sesame oil**
  THERAPEUTIC ACTION: Builds all seven skin layers
  PREPARATION METHOD: Rub skin with sesame oil
- **Turnips**
  THERAPEUTIC ACTION: Cleanses skin; relieves acne and eczema
  PREPARATION METHOD: Vegetable compress

SLEEP DISORDERS

TEACHING

Sleep is a natural rhythm of the body. Good sleep patterns are important because they support the other deep rhythms of the body such as breathing, digestion, and heartbeat. Sleep brings the rhythm of the cosmos into our biological life. During the day, our system is in a *receptive* mode, receiving the input of energies from the planets, the sun, and star systems. During the night, we are also open to these cosmic influences, but in a *giving* mode, where the energies of our biological processes are returned to the cosmos to share in all other activities of the universe. Furthermore, sleep is not just a time of rest, for we can rest without sleeping—it is a time when the body, mind, and spirit integrate all that we have experienced during the last twenty-four hours.

The Biological Function of Sleep

The body prepares us for sleep not through our habits but through its biological functions. Two primary functions create our sleep mode. Around 8 P.M., the body's nerve system switches from the sympathetic mode, which stimulates us to perform work and activities, to the parasympathetic mode, which calms and soothes our systems and moves us from a state of outer awareness to a state of inner awareness. At this time, the body begins to rest and prepare for sleep.

Each of the body's main organs works with a partner and each organ pair represents a particular functional system. Each organ in the pair is most active during roughly a two-hour time span within the day's twenty-four-hour cycle. The body functions by way of this organ clock. From 10:30 P.M. to 3 A.M., the time for natural sleep, the Liver/Gallbladder System operates at its peak function. The Liver/Gallbladder pair is a metabolic system that deals with the final stages of food digestion as well as the digestion of the impressions and emotional experiences we have had throughout that day. The Liver/Gallbladder System relates to the energy of space, which creates a place or "space" for renewal so that all things can be thoroughly digested and integrated into our minds and bodies.

If we don't follow the natural rhythm of sleep and, for example, habitually stay up late working or eating a late-night meal, the body is forced to remain in its active mode. As a result, the last stages of both physical and emotional digestion will not be fully completed. This incomplete digestion will cause long-term problems for the up-building processes of the mind and body, creating imbalances and deficiencies that can only be avoided by bringing the body back to its normal sleep rhythms.

Exceptions that occur once in a while, like eating after 8 P.M. or staying up late, is never a real problem as long as it doesn't become a habit. We are accustomed to making work and social activities the highest priority in our daily life, but when habits interfere with our bodily functions and health, we need to reconsider our lifestyle.

Good sleep patterns are so vital for the body and mind that we often need to learn how to prepare for sleep. Ingesting food or experiencing strong emotional stimulants like television or films close to bedtime will ultimately disrupt our sleep patterns. These activities, which are okay in themselves, require the daytime functions of our body and mind in order to be digested and integrated properly. When done at bedtime, they disturb the body and mind's natural preparations for sleep. These nonintegrated areas will become like toxins that do not nourish the body but inhibit all of its deeper functions.

Sleep and Consciousness

When sleeping, the body changes the mode of its consciousness, but remains awake and receives all the inputs from its immediate environment. Bedrooms should be painted with passive, soothing pastel colors in the bluish range, rather than in the stimulating heated colors like the reds, yellows, and oranges. The mind should find rest through affirmations—prayer or meditation to calm and still the mind's activities can be done just prior to going to sleep.

Falling to sleep is a process that is deeply psychological as well as physical.

To fall asleep, we need to release our sense of conscious control that we feel we have over life while awake and active. When feelings of insecurity consciously or unconsciously influence us, we perceive life as being somewhat threatening. When we feel unable to control life, we unconsciously resist the letting go required to enter into sleep. This inability to "let go" is not so much an emotional problem, though there can be emotional symptoms, but a spiritual issue. Only our spiritual nature can understand life as beautiful, secure, and nonthreatening, regardless of the circumstantial events of life, some of which can be very trying. Sleep is our way of surrendering to the goodness of life and ultimately trusting in its process.

Quiet time for children, and being together with those they love just before they sleep, is very important. Before giving themselves to sleep, children need to know and experience that all is well in their world, that they are safe and loved. A child who has unresolved conflicts or fears will not sleep well and, if this situation persists, it will influence their development and well-being. Prayer or affirming, calming words are important for a child, especially if presented as a little bedtime ceremony or ritual that involves the child interactively.

All cultures respond to the great movements of life with the solemnity of prayer and ceremony. Such rituals are acts of love, trust, and thanksgiving, the foundation of the experience of life practiced in all religions and spiritual paths. The time set aside for focusing on love and trust are profound and healthy ways of recognizing the deep cycles of life—birth and birthdays, marriage, death, and sleep, when we relinquish our conscious sense of control to the fullness of our dreams.

THERAPY

INSOMNIA

Remedy #1
- 1 cup of milk
- $\frac{1}{4}$ teaspoon nutmeg
- $\frac{1}{8}$ teaspoon honey

To warm milk, add the nutmeg powder and the honey. Drink before bedtime.

Remedy #2
- Sesame oil

Massage the soles of the feet and crown of the head with warm sesame oil.

Remedy #3
- 6–8 chamomile buds
- 1 cup boiling water

To prepare tea, steep chamomile buds in boiling water. Drink before bedtime.

Remedy #4
- $\frac{1}{2}$ teaspoon cinnamon powder
- 1 cup boiling water
- Honey

To prepare a tea, mix the cinnamon in boiling water. Simmer with lid on for 5 minutes. Sweeten with a little honey. Drink 1 cup 2 times per day.

Tissue Salts

- *Natrum mur.* 6X
- *Mag. phos.* 6X
- *Calc. phos.* 6X

Take these remedies together just before bedtime for up to two weeks.

UNREFRESHING SLEEP

Tissue Salts

- *Natrum mur.* 6X

Take 1 dose before bedtime and 1 dose upon waking in the morning. Repeat for up to two weeks.

GENERAL PROMOTION OF SLEEP

Spices, Herbs, and Foods

- **Chamomile**

  THERAPEUTIC ACTION: Alleviates insomnia

  PREPARATION METHOD: Herbal bath—Pour 1 quart of boiling water over 3 teaspoons of dried chamomile or 2 chamomile teabags; let steep 10 minutes, pour into bath water, and soak for 15 minutes. Tea—Place 10 chamomile buds in 1 cup of water; pour boiling water over them and let steep for 5 minutes; drink 1 hour before bedtime.

- **Cloves**

  THERAPEUTIC ACTION: Alleviates insomnia

  PREPARATION METHOD: Bruise 1 teaspoon of cloves and add 4 teaspoons of water. Slowly simmer in a covered pan for 8 minutes. Add 1 teaspoon of liquid to 6 ounces of water and take at bedtime.

- **Dill**
  THERAPEUTIC ACTION: Induces sleep
  PREPARATION METHOD: Place a sprig of fresh dill near the pillow.
- **Pumpkin seeds**
  THERAPEUTIC ACTION: Alleviates insomnia
  PREPARATION METHOD: Include in the daily diet

Reflexology

For instructions on reflexology, see "Reflexology" under "How to Use the Therapy Section" at the beginning of Part II.

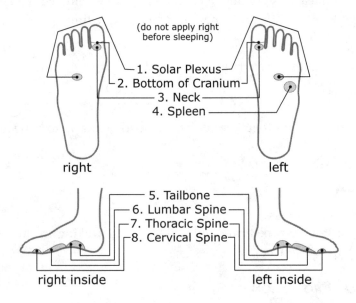

(do not apply right before sleeping)
1. Solar Plexus
2. Bottom of Cranium
3. Neck
4. Spleen

right   left

5. Tailbone
6. Lumbar Spine
7. Thoracic Spine
8. Cervical Spine

right inside   left inside

URINARY SYSTEM DIFFICULTIES

TEACHING

Among the body's organ systems, the Kidney/Bladder System is unique because it is the foundation of all the prebirth and postbirth functional energies at work in the body's tissues and cells. The Kidney/Bladder System is like an invisible umbilical cord reaching into our past and connecting our hereditary patterns to our present life. Yet, it continually creates the basis for our future. In the Chinese medical concept, the kidneys control "the Fire of the Gate of Life." This phrase is a rather beautiful and poetic way of saying that the kidneys control the basis of all cell metabolism and mediate the fundamental functional energies of all organ systems.

As in all other tissue systems, any factors that compromise the Kidney/Bladder System and the reproductive organs, such as hormone replacement therapy, drug side effects, IUDs, and surgery, can create immune reactions and symptoms in both the kidneys and bladder.

Embryological Development of the Kidneys

The Kidney/Bladder System develops from the embryological tissue called the mesoderm, the same tissue that develops the heart and reproductive organs. Thus, the kidneys and bladder are connected anatomically and energetically to these very important organ systems. This connection proves significant because the Kidney/Bladder System controls the process of insemination and fertility, which relates to the ability to conceive a new child through the reproductive organs. At the moment of conception, two important energy patterns controlled by the kidneys merge and begin their mutual work together: the pattern of *hereditary* energies that we inherit through our genes and the pattern of *functional* energies that energize all of the body's emerging systems and tissues.

The Kidney/Bladder System not only facilitates the conception of new offspring but also gives new birth to our systems, cells, and tissues on a daily basis. Thousands of cells die daily and are replaced by the birth of new ones. In fact, every twenty-four hours, our body reproduces itself. Living organisms are not like machines—running until their parts give out or they need more fuel. Organisms live through the life energies metabolized by their tissue systems. The biological clocks that determine the functions of these systems work on "sun" and "star" time. We can observe this clock as we watch the progression of the star constellations moving across the night horizon, or the light and shadows following the sun from dawn to dark, or the seasons changing. The biological clock of the body begins and ends its cycle at 3 A.M., starting with the life-giving Lung System. It moves in two-hour segments through all the systems and ends with the Liver System, which has completed its metabolic integration of the whole twenty-four-hour cycle. Just as the first independent breath of the newborn infant signifies new life, so the Lung System resets the biological clock anew every twenty-four hours, renewing us, recreating life in the functions of our cells and tissues, and making new experiences possible.

The Kidneys and Our Psychology

The kidneys also play a major role in our psychological makeup. They have much to do with our emotions, especially the stress patterns that produce nervousness, fear, and anxiety, all of which are kidney "responses." In addition, the kidneys relate to our nerve and sensory systems. Stress energies from these systems are "drying" energies—we see kidney involvement in situations in which anxiety and nervousness lead to frequent or uncontrolled urination.

When we feel anxious, we also notice that our breathing patterns change. The kidneys actually control the breathing function of the lungs by providing for the lungs' ability to metabolize air. The lungs develop from the same embryological tissue, the endoderm, as our intestinal tract and it is the ingested and "digested" air we breathe that is part of the nutrition of our cells and tissues. The hereditary and functional energies of the kidneys not only support the lungs in this nutritive process, but play a major role in all of the body's metabolic functions, without which digestion would be impossible.

The lungs are also part of a rhythm system that, along with the heart, helps stabilize and integrate all mind and body functions. The heart's rhythmical beating corresponds to the rhythm of the lungs breathing in and out. The heart is the major organ of our rhythm system and is connected directly to the kidney functions. Hence, the kidneys, along with the lungs and the heart, all mesodermic organs, play a major role in the rhythmic functions of the body and mind.

The Kidney and Body Functions

The kidneys control other physiological functions within the body. Their metabolic energies control the physiological function of the brain and nerve tissues, as well as the bones. In addition, our sense of hearing depends on the kidneys. Hearing is accomplished by signals from nerve tissues stimulated by the bony structures in our middle and inner ear. These nerve tissues extend into brain centers that reproduce them as sounds. Again, all of these nerve and brain tissues are controlled by the kidney.

The kidney and bladder, though partners in a single system, have different functions. We might say that the kidney contains and creates functional energies and the bladder carries and disperses these energies throughout the body. One of the most important of these energies is what Classical medicine calls "primary immune energy," which also can be called "basic immunity." This energy of the immune system works in all cells and tissues of the body.

Immune energy is created by the Kidney/Bladder System and the reproductive organs working together and is transported from its storage in the kidneys throughout the body by the kidney's partner, the bladder.

The bladder, of course, has other jobs. It stores the urine processed in the kidneys and controls the function of urination. The body's fluids are products of metabolic processes occurring in cells and tissues and these fluids undergo their main refining in the kidneys. The kidneys filter out the byproducts of cell metabolism, which eventually become urine. Then, they reabsorb, transform, and energize the refined fluid for further use. Urine is therefore actually a "mirror" of all the processes occurring in the body and mind. In Classical medicine, urine analysis and urine diagnosis are used for accurately evaluating the health status of patients. Because urine contains all of the byproducts of the metabolic processes taking place in the body, it has been used as a therapeutic substance in Classical medicine, European naturopathic medicine, and homeopathy.

THERAPY

BLADDER/KIDNEY INFECTIONS

The symptom of a possible kidney infection is usually pain in a localized area below the rib cage at the upper end of the small of the back; this pain can also be due to stones in the kidney. If you experience this symptom, consult your natural healthcare professional.

Frequent urination during the day and night, but unaccompanied by other bladder symptoms, could be a symptom of diabetes or, in men, of prostate enlargement and should also be evaluated by a natural healthcare professional. Frequent urination with other symptoms, such as pain in the bladder, or a feeling of burning or irritation upon urination and discolored or smelly urine, is a sign of an immune reaction in the bladder. The outer tissues of the bladder are mucous membranes that can become inflamed as they react to any factor affecting the bladder itself or to toxins in the urine.

As in all other cases in which membranes are involved, taking antibiotics only kills the bacteria and does not address the true cause of the symptoms. Remember, the presence of bacteria is part of the immune reaction; the bacteria are not the cause of the problem but a response to factors that are compromising the tissues. By helping the body overcome the symptoms naturally, the tissues become stronger and more skillful in their functions and the immune system "program" is strengthened for any future need.

General Remedies

Remedy #1

- Parsley
- 1 cup boiling water

Pour boiling water over a small handful of parsley leaves and stems. Steep for 5 minutes with a lid on the cup. Drink 3 times per day.

Remedy #2

- Cranberry juice (pure organic), or cranberry capsules

Drink 6 ounces of cranberry juice, or take cranberry capsules (dosage recommended on the bottle) 4 times per day.

Remedy #3

- Barley
- Water

Mix 1 part barley with 4 parts water. Boil gently in a pan (with the lid on) for 20 minutes. Strain and drink 1 cup 2–3 times per day for up to five days.

Tissue Salts

- *Ferrum phos.* 6X
- *Kali mur.* 6X
- *Natrum mur.* 6X
- *Calc. sulph.* 6X
- *Natrum sulph.* 6X

Take these remedies together 4–5 times daily for up to four days. Reduce the number of doses as symptoms begin to improve.

Spices, Herbs, and Foods

- **Asparagus**
  PREPARATION METHOD: Include in the daily diet
- **Fennel seed**
  PREPARATION METHOD: Standard hot infusion, decoction, dry plant tincture
- **Chicory**
  PREPARATION METHOD: Decoction, fresh plant tincture
- **Corn silk** (from corn cob)
  PREPARATION METHOD: Simmer a large handful of corn silk in 1 quart of water for 10 minutes. Strain liquid. Drink 1–2 glasses of liquid daily.
- **Cranberry juice** (pure organic)
  PREPARATION METHOD: Include in the daily diet

KIDNEY STONES

Stones that form in the gallbladder, bladder, or kidneys are composed of insoluble organic substances that result from impaired and incomplete metabolic processes in the primary digestive organs. Stones can create symptoms in the kidneys and bladder. See your natural healthcare professional for evaluation.

Tissue Salts

- *Calc. phos.* 6X
- *Mag. phos.* 6X
- *Natrum sulph.* 6X
- *Silicea* 6X
  Take these remedies together 3 times per day for up to three weeks.

Spices, Herbs, and Foods

- **Asparagus**
  PREPARATION METHOD: Include in the daily diet
- **Fennel seed**
  PREPARATION METHOD: Standard hot infusion, decoction, dry plant tincture
- **Celery**
  PREPARATION METHOD: Decoction
- **Chicory**
  PREPARATION METHOD: Decoction, fresh plant tincture
- **Cranberry juice** (pure organic)
  PREPARATION METHOD: Include in the daily diet

GENERAL CARE OF THE URINARY SYSTEM

Spices, Herbs, and Foods

- **Asparagus**
  THERAPEUTIC ACTION: Softens stones; relieves edema, obstructed urination, bladder irritation, and cystitis
  PREPARATION METHOD: Include in the daily diet
- **Celery**
  THERAPEUTIC ACTION: Helps reduce kidney stones; relieves cystitis and nephritis; diuretic action
  PREPARATION METHOD: Decoction
- **Chicory**
  THERAPEUTIC ACTION: Relieves painful urination and cystitis; helps reduce urinary stones

PREPARATION METHOD: Decoction, fresh plant tincture
- **Corn**

    THERAPEUTIC ACTION: Helps reduce kidney stones

    PREPARATION METHOD: Include in the daily diet
- **Corn silk** (from corn cob)

    THERAPEUTIC ACTION: Helps pass urine; relieves edema

    PREPARATION METHOD: Simmer a large handful of corn silk in 1 quart of water for 10 minutes. Strain liquid. Drink 1–2 glasses of liquid daily.
- **Cranberry juice** (pure organic)

    THERAPEUTIC ACTION: Helps reduce kidney stones; relieves cystitis; helps support kidney function

    PREPARATION METHOD: Include in the daily diet
- **Fennel seed**

    THERAPEUTIC ACTION: Helps reduce kidney stones; relieves irritated bladder; restores urinary system

    PREPARATION METHOD: Standard hot infusion, decoction, dry plant tincture
- **Parsley**

    THERAPEUTIC ACTION: Acts as a diuretic; relieves cystitis and kidney inflammation

    PREPARATION METHOD: Decoction, fresh plant tincture

Reflexology

For instructions on reflexology, see "Reflexology" under "How to Use the Therapy Section" at the beginning of Part II.

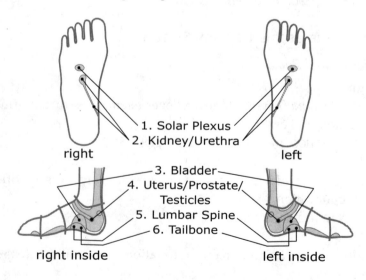

right   left

1. Solar Plexus
2. Kidney/Urethra
3. Bladder
4. Uterus/Prostate/ Testicles
5. Lumbar Spine
6. Tailbone

right inside   left inside

PART THREE

The Therapeutic Nature of Foods

The Nature and Nutritional Effects of Common Foods

Western medical science bases its understanding of biological processes on what can be weighed and measured. A discussion of nutrition from this viewpoint centers on the substances found in our foods, such as minerals, vitamins, and proteins. All of these substances, which conventional medicine calls nutrients, are first and foremost the products of inner biological transformations that result from energetic, not chemical, processes. In other words, the biochemicals, proteins, minerals, and vitamins found in the body are all created by the energies of metabolism. In this sense, all nutrients are products of, not the cause of, nutrition.

Because all the energetic functions of the body and mind are involved in the process of digestion, they provide the basis for nutrition. Remember that the body and mind function by way of integrated organ systems. Each system has its own energetic components that play major roles in the way the body and mind digest nutrients and nourish themselves.

Digestion is composed of two processes. The catabolic process breaks down components in the food we eat. This process is similar to starting a fire to get warm: as the wood burns, becoming ash, it releases the warmth and light we need. Likewise, the food we ingest needs to be "burned" in the digestive fire in order to make the energy of the food's nutrients available for further processing. Our bodies then use the energy released to create new nutrient substances. This phase, which builds the cells and tissues of the body, is called the anabolic stage of metabolism.

Each of the major tissue groups in the body has its own form of digestive activities that include catabolic and anabolic processes. In the course of completing these processes, each tissue system retains certain nutrients for itself and passes the rest on to the next tissue group. The energetic process of digestion begins in the Stomach System, which controls the lymphatic processes as well as sugar and carbohydrate metabolism. The process then proceeds to the Blood System, then, progressively, to the Muscle System, the Fat Tissue System, the Bone Tissue System, the Bone/Nerve System, and finally, to the tissues of the Reproductive Organ System. The end products of this cycle of digestion nourish all the cells, the basic immunity and the primary biological energies that control our systems. The whole process takes about ten days for the body to fully complete.

NUTRITIONAL ENERGIES

The Classical medical sciences do not describe foods by the vitamins, proteins, or minerals they contain but by their *nutritive energy components* and how these energies affect the functions of the body and mind. In this sense, it is a much more reliable system for understanding the nature of foods than merely stating what nutrients they contain. This is because the life functions of the body and mind are based on energy and not on substances. At death, what was once a living organism still contains all the nutrient and biochemical substances it had, but the vital energies that govern and determine the life and function of the organism are gone.

Classical medicine divides foods into metabolic groups called *Tastes*. This term refers not only to how a food tastes in the mouth, but more important, it identifies the *energetic* components found in each food group, as well. Each energy component associated with a particular Taste has specific effects on the body and mind and makes up the complex process we call nutrition. The energy components of each Taste are defined as either catabolic or anabolic and either cooling or heating. In addition, each Taste is composed of two of the major energetic Elements that influence the functions of the body and mind. Most foods are made up of two or more Tastes. The ones mentioned below are used to illustrate the concept of Taste because they reflect the main actions and components reviewed in each category. The name of the Taste is followed by its effect on the digestive metabolism and the Elements to which it belongs.

By better understanding the energy effects of the six Taste groups, you can learn to adjust your diet to fit temporary, immediate needs. There can be times of stress, for example, when you would need more of the Sweet Taste than Bitter or Pungent. The best general rule for the daily diet is to include at least one food of each Taste in each meal to get the full spectrum of food energies.

Sweet Taste (Anabolic–Cooling)/Earth and Water Elements

- Decreases stress in the nerve system
- Decreases enzymatic activity
- Increases a sense of well-being and groundedness
- Increases cell and the building up of tissues
- Increases wholesomeness to the body
- Increases fluids, blood tissues, and immunity
- Provides strength
- Stimulates immune system
- Nourishes and soothes the body and mind

In Excess:

- Creates obesity, lethargy and heaviness
- Increases mucus
- Increases blood sugar levels and promotes diabetes

Examples of Sweet Taste

Rice, wheat, cane sugar, milk, ghee, butter, coconut, coconut oil, figs, purple grapes, melons, black lentils, garbanzo beans, mung beans, cucumber, beets, almonds, sunflower oil, maple syrup, and cashews.

Sour Taste (Anabolic–Heating)/Earth and Fire Elements

- Decreases stress in the nerve system
- Increases a sense of groundedness
- Increases enzymatic activity and salivation
- Stimulates appetite
- Strengthens the mind
- Sharpens the senses

In Excess:

- Increases thirst

- Increases mucus

- Creates toxins in the blood

- Promotes edema, heartburn, and high acidity

Examples of Sour Taste

Cheese, yogurt, rose hips, lemon, oranges, and green grapes.

Salt Taste (Anabolic–Heating)/Water and Fire Elements

- Decreases stress in the nerve system

- Increases enzymatic activity

- Increases sense of groundedness

- Aids digestion

- Helps control spasms and cramps

- Acts as a laxative

- Aids salivation

- Retains fluids

- Inhibits actions of all other Tastes

In Excess:

- Disturbs blood tissue

- Increases heat and inflammation in the body

- Increases skin symptoms

- Promotes gastric ulcers and gastric inflammation

- Increases blood pressure

Examples of Salt Taste

Sea salt, rock salt, and kelp.

Pungent Taste (Catabolic–Heating)/Air and Fire Elements

- Decreases mucus
- Decreases sense of groundedness
- Increases nerve responses
- Increases enzymatic activity
- Promotes digestion and food absorption
- Helps food metabolism
- Cleanses blood tissues
- Relieves skin problems
- Helps eliminate blood clots
- Cleanses bodily tissues

In Excess:

- Increases heat in the body
- Promotes abnormal sweating
- Creates burning sensations and irritation in gastric and heart areas
- Promotes dizziness

Examples of Pungent Taste

Onion, radish, chili, ginger, garlic, cumin, cayenne pepper, white mustard oil, mustard seed, black pepper, celery seed, and clove.

Bitter Taste (Catabolic–Cooling)/Air and Space Elements

- Decreases enzymatic activity
- Decreases sense of groundedness
- Increases nerve responses
- Strengthens all other Tastes
- Antibiotic and germicidal
- Helps control dizziness and fainting

In Excess:

- Causes burning or itching sensations
- Dries skin and tissues
- Reduces functions of the bone marrow and sperm
- Causes "ungrounded" sensations

Examples of Bitter Taste

Rhubarb, dandelion root, fenugreek, and osha.

Astringent Taste (Catabolic–Cooling)/Air and Earth Elements

- Decreases enzymatic activity
- Decreases sense of groundedness
- Increases nerve responses
- Acts as a sedative
- Increases blood coagulation
- Constricts blood vessels
- Anti-inflammatory

In Excess:

- Creates dryness of the mouth
- Constipating
- Inhibits heart functions

Examples of Astringent Taste

Unripe banana, barley, goat's milk, cabbage, cauliflower, celery, lettuce, potato, apple, pears, and pomegranates.

Special Diets

Special diets making claims about the health benefits of their protocols are very popular today. It can be confusing that new diet regimens appear all the time and that the whole field of nutrition seems to change its mind radically every year or so. What was "in" and healthy one year is now "out" and unhealthy the next.

Humans were created to eat a broad range of foods in order to maintain health. This is because each food substance has its own particular nutritive energies and qualities that nourish specific needs in our cells and tissues. Whenever we limit our daily nutrition through specialty diets, we are narrowing the scope of our nutritional metabolic elements—if we continue with these diets, we end up malnourished and our cell and tissue functions suffer.

In natural medicine, diet is an important part of the health protocols. In some cases, therapeutic diets that restrict some foods and increase the use of others are prescribed in order to reestablish the health of the body. These diets are, however, used only for short periods of time, and as soon as they have achieved their purpose, the patient is returned to a normal, all-inclusive diet. Therapeutic diets should only be prescribed by a natural healthcare professional to avoid compromising your nutrition.

One of the most prevalent departures from a normal diet is vegetarianism. Eliminating animal products from one's diet is used to a certain degree in all cultures, though for different reasons. In the Eastern and Middle Eastern traditions, vegetarianism is used in connection with spiritual practices or as a therapy. Some Western traditions claim that vegetarianism is the only way to maintain good health and that we were not made to eat meat. This is not true. Animal products come from an entirely different biological kingdom than plants. The plant kingdom and the animal kingdom contain unique forms of nutrient potentials and metabolic energies. It is incorrect to say that animal proteins can be substituted for plant proteins—their respective metabolic energies and how they support and nourish the body and mind are very different. If we have generally good health and don't need to be on a specially prescribed therapeutic diet, we need the nutrients from both sources to maintain health.

The only two justifications for a vegetarian diet are in connection with a spiritual belief system or practice (in which the focus is not on the nutritional aspects of a diet but on a particular spiritual perspective) or as a short-term dietary change prescribed as part of a therapeutic process. It is interesting to note that in Hinduism and Buddhism, where vegetarianism is a usual part of their spiritual practice, whenever one becomes ill, the natural doctor often prescribes meat and animal products to be used therapeutically to restore health.

THE USE OF SUPPLEMENTS

Another myth in Western health practices is that we need vitamin and mineral supplements in order to be healthy. This concept reflects a misunderstanding of what nutrients are and how our digestion metabolizes them. All the natural nutrients our body needs to maintain its health are found in foods. The nutrients in a carrot, for instance, are bound in a very complex relationship to all the cells and tissues in the whole carrot. This relationship of biochemical and energetic components is the real nutrition of the carrot, not its separate ingredients. If we extract vitamin A (beta-carotene) from the carrot and take it as a supplement, the vitamin A is no longer a part of the relationship of elements that makes it truly effective.

Classical medicine uses whole food supplements. This means that if you need extra vitamin A, for example, you make carrot juice (with the pulp), increasing your intake of a food that contains vitamin A but without compromising the effective relationships that determine how the vitamin will be used by the body.

The body is programmed to respond correctly only to things that are found in nature—there is no such thing as a "vitamin A tree." When we extract substances from nature, we compromise the way we digest and utilize the nutrients. When our systems encounter unnatural substances like extracted vitamins and minerals, the immune system must activate in order to integrate the "foreign" nature of the substances and our digestion has to alter its normal procedures to deal with them. The net result is poorer, rather than greater, health.

The only exception to this is working with terminally ill (dying) patients.

When the body is no longer capable of supporting its vital processes or reestablishing their normal functions, intervention in the natural processes may be necessary to enhance the quality of life. In this special circumstance, nutrients that are no longer being digested properly can be introduced directly into the blood as supplements in order to help stabilize the weakened biological processes.

HEALTHY EATING

Our nutritional health is based on the quality of the food we eat, how we combine and prepare it, and how healthy our digestive system is. Nonorganic foods contain toxins, are denatured, and no longer contain the biological vitality that is essential for our digestive processes. Genetically engineered foods should always be avoided! The use of microwave cooking devices destroys the vital energies of even organic foods and should also be avoided.

Another important aspect of healthy eating is what we could call the start-

A Word about Water

We often forget that water is not just H_2O but a living nutrient essential for our health and well-being. Rainwater, the original source of our drinking water, is distilled through the process of evaporation and condensation. As rain falls, it seeps into the ground, flowing through the vast mineral and metal deposits of the earth, while water from melting snow fields and glaciers also carves deep into the earth. The water from these sources slowly becomes potent with powerful earth energies. When this process is complete, the energized water makes its way to the surface as a spring. The water flowing from springs is the source of our rivers. You notice that rivers bend and curve in a figure eight as they move through our landscapes. This universal pattern of movement is not due to the nature of the landscape itself, such as soil or rock formations, but is a result of the living energy in the water. Spring water contains the same energy of the earth and heavens that our bodies need as part of their essential nutrients.

Distilled water, reverse osmosis, and processed water lack this essential nutritive quality. This is doubly problematic in that it is the nature of water to gather and retain energies. Just as water gathers energies and substances from the earth in order to restore its living properties, so denatured water will consume energy and substances from our systems in order to restore itself.

ing and stopping of the digestive process. The Sweet Taste always starts the basic digestive processes and therefore should be used at the beginning of a meal. This is not like eating a heavy dessert as a first course, but pertains to using foods with the Sweet Taste energies, like rice and wheat. Often in Eastern and Middle Eastern cuisines, a pinch of cane sugar is added to first course dishes. Conversely, it's the energies of the Bitter Taste foods that "close" the digestive processes so that the food you've eaten can be further metabolized without interference. Foods like green salads or a green tea contain bitter energies. In American culture, we usually reverse these important nutritional concepts by eating a salad as a first course and ending with a heavy, sweet dessert—and then we wonder why indigestion seems to be so common.

Drinking while eating also represses the digestive processes by diluting enzymes and digestive fluids that are important for the metabolism. Consuming cold drinks is even worse because digestive processes are "hot" processes; the cold drinks cool down the digestive activity and prevent complete metabolism of foods, leading to a buildup of digestive toxins and resulting in impaired nutrition.

COMBINING FOODS

Digestive metabolism is governed by energies rather than by chemistry. All of the biochemicals in our digestive process are produced by the energies inherent in our food, water, and the air we breathe. In the Classical medical traditions, these energies are referred to as "Tastes" (Sweet, Sour, Salt, Pungent, Bitter, Astringent). Everything in nature is composed of varying combinations of the Elements of Earth, Water, Fire, Air, and Space. These Elements influence all our tissues and their processes. For example, the predominance of the Water and Fire Elements produces the Salt Taste; salt itself is made up primarily of these two energies. Conversely, a predominance of Water and Earth energies will produce the Sweet Taste, of which sugar is a good example. Our digestion unlocks these energies in foods. This unlocking of and utilization of energies defines the process of nutrition.

All foods fall into categories of metabolic energies, but these energies are not always compatible with one another (see Digestive Dysfunction in Part Two). Learning to combine foods correctly plays as important a role in nutrition as eating "healthy" foods. Foods that are improperly combined in the same meal will tend to produce toxins and inhibit the digestive process. Here is a list that will help you avoid errors in food combining.

Milk does not combine well with bananas, fish, melons, yogurt, sour fruits, kitchari (for those following an Ayurvedic diet), yeast breads, or red meat

Yogurt does not combine well with milk, sour fruits, melons, hot drinks, fish, mango, starches, cheese, or bananas

Eggs do not combine well with milk, yogurt, cheese, fruits, or potatoes

Melons do not combine well with any other foods

Honey does not combine well with ghee or grains

Lemons do not combine well with yogurt, milk, cucumber, or tomato

Starches do not combine well with bananas, eggs, milk, or dates

Corn does not combine well with dates, raisins, or bananas

Nightshades (potato, tomato, eggplant) do not combine well with yogurt, milk, or cucumber

BALANCING THE ENERGIES OF FOOD WITH SPICES AND HERBS

All foods are made up of specific energy patterns that determine their nutritional value and the way we digest them (see The Nature and Nutritional Effects of Common Foods, on pages 263–268). Foods usually contain much more of one type of metabolic energy than another, but using spices will balance these energies. Eastern and Middle Eastern diets have always used spices or herbs to balance the energies in foods and enhance their digestive properties. Here are some suggestions from these traditions and from their European counterparts. The following foods can be balanced by using the spices or herbs indicated. Use the spices or herbs during the same meal, even if they are in another dish, or season the particular food with one or more of the recommended spices or herbs.

Dairy

Cheese can be balanced by using cayenne pepper, black pepper, chili pepper, or fennel

Ice cream can be balanced by using black pepper, cloves, or cardamom

Sour cream can be balanced by using coriander, cardamom, rosemary, thyme, or fennel

Yogurt can be balanced by using black pepper, ginger, cumin, or rosemary

Eggs can be balanced by using turmeric, cilantro, onions, parsley, or sage

Vegetables

Beans and peas can be balanced by using cloves, garlic, black pepper, ginger, chili, fennel, rosemary, oregano, or rock salt

Cabbage can be balanced by using turmeric, mustard seed, fennel, or rosemary

Green salad can be balanced by using lemon juice, olive oil, fennel, oregano, or rosemary

Onion can be balanced by using lemon, mustard seed, fennel

Potato can be balanced by using clarified butter, black pepper, rosemary, fennel, or thyme

Tomato can be balanced by using cumin, lime, oregano, fennel, rosemary, or thyme

Meat and Fish

Fish can be balanced by using lemon, lime, or coconut

Red meats can be balanced by using chili, cayenne, cloves, fennel, oregano, or rosemary

Grains

Oats can be balanced by using mustard seed, turmeric, cumin, or fennel

Rice can be balanced by using black pepper, cloves, cinnamon, cardamom, fennel, or rosemary

Wheat can be balanced by using ginger, black pepper, fennel, or rosemary

Seeds and Nuts

Nuts (all) can be balanced by soaking overnight and then frying with olive oil, chili, or fennel

Seeds (all) can be balanced by soaking overnight then cooking or baking with sage or oregano

Fruits

Banana can be balanced by using cardamom or black pepper

Melon can be balanced by using coriander or coconut meat

Watermelon can be balanced by using rock salt or chili

Dried fruits can be balanced by soaking in water overnight

Other

Black tea can be balanced by using ginger or cinnamon

Coffee can be balanced by using cardamom (plus nutmeg if overstimulation occurs from drinking coffee)

Chocolate can be balanced by using cumin or cardamom

Sweets and sugars can be balanced by using ginger, fennel, or rosemary

DIETS FOR SPECIFIC HEALTH ISSUES

You may have health issues that are beyond the scope of this book in terms of specific therapies. Whether you are following other procedures in natural health care or are under treatment by a conventional medical doctor, the following dietary suggestions will help support your health and will not interfere with other treatments. All foods should be organically grown and not prepared using a microwave. Good foods are listed in plain type; very good foods in *italics;* and especially good foods in **boldface.**

Arteriosclerosis and Cholesterol Control Diet

Vegetables—**Mung beans**, *beans, lentils, radish*, **onion**, *leeks, garlic*, chives, leafy greens, *cabbage, spinach*, **carrots with greens**, *kale, broccoli, parsley*, **asparagus**, *red or green bell peppers, tomato, celery*, cucumber, *hot peppers, peas*, **avocados**, sprouts

Fruits—**Apples**, *grapefruit*, oranges, apricots, mangoes, grapes, *banana*, pineapple

Fish—*Sardines, salmon, mackerel, tuna, herring*

Nuts—**Almond**, *hazelnut, pumpkin seed*, **walnut**

Grains—**Amaranth**, *buckwheat, barley*, **rye, oats/oat bran, quinoa**

Other—*Mint leaf, seaweed, chlorella, shiitake mushrooms, rose hips, horseradish*, **olive oil, grape seed oil, red wine, green or black tea**, flaxseeds, flaxseed oil, *dandelion greens, bee pollen*

Spices and Herbs—*Hawthorne berry, dandelion root, burdock root, chaparral*, peppermint. **cayenne pepper, ginger**, rhubarb root, yarrow, chamomile, motherwort, valerian, **cloves, Irish moss**

Plaque Reduction

Bilberry, **garlic**, L-carnitine, coenzyme Q_{10}, hawthorn (as an herb), ginger, alfalfa, blueberries, omega-3 fatty acids from fish oil, grapefruit pulp/membranes, chlorella

Avoid—Excess animal fats; excess amounts of cheese and whole milk; poultry skin; corn and safflower oil; margarine; processed foods

AntiCancer Diet

Reduction of Chemotherapy Effects and Radiation

Hijiki/wakame/kelp seaweeds, wheat/barley grass supplements, *fennel seed* (chewed or prepared as tea), *astragalus herb, aloe vera juice or gel,* shark cartilage

Prevention and Treatment

Garlic (for immune system enhancement—Peel 30 cloves of garlic and let them rest 15 minutes before further handling. Place in a blender or food processor, add a small amount of water, and blend using short bursts until homogenized. Add 1 part homogenized garlic to 20 parts water; drink two glasses a day. Refrigerate garlic for further use.

Vegetables—Garlic, **cabbage**, onions, carrots, tomatoes, broccoli, collard greens, sweet potatoes, kale, beans, cauliflower, any dark-green leafy vegetable, any yellow-orange fruit or vegetable, sprouts, beets, radish, asparagus, **brussels sprouts**, turnip, cucumber (with peel), **broccoli, bok choy**

Fruits—All citrus fruits, *apricots*, peaches, *red grapes*; eat no fruits in the same meal with other foods, except meals or snacks consisting of only grains

Fish—*Mackerel,* salmon, sardines, herring, pilchard

Nuts—Brazil nuts, walnuts, almonds

Grains—Oats, rye, groats (kasha), barley, amaranth

Spices and Herbs—Anise, dill, **fennel**, coriander, marjoram, *ginger,* sage, saffron, thyme, *rosemary,* bay leaf, sorrel, **turmeric**, mint, oregano, basil

Other—*Green tea,* licorice root, wheat bran, shiitake/ling zhi (reishi)/ maitake mushrooms, yogurt, olive oil, acidophilus milk products, kelp/ hijiki/wakame seaweeds, wheat/barley grass, chlorella.

Avoid—Red meats, standard vegetable oils/margarines, excessive alcohol, excess salt

Diabetes Diet

Vegetables—**Raw and boiled onion, garlic, sautéed mushrooms, cabbage, lettuce, turnips, beans, broccoli, alfalfa, mung beans, lentils, kidney beans, asparagus, watercress**

Fruits—Rhubarb

Grains—Barley

Spices—Fenugreek, **cinnamon**, black pepper, dry ginger, long pepper (*Piper longum*), bay leaf, cardamom, mustard seed, cumin, turmeric

Prohibited Foods—Rice, potato, sweet potato, carrots, milk, parsnips, beetroot, bananas, raisins, candy, sugars

Daily Regimen:

1. Swallow 7 black peppercorns whole with water each morning.

2. Mix 1 portion of organic cottage cheese, 1 tablespoon of organic flaxseed oil, and $\frac{1}{8}$ teaspoon of cayenne pepper or turmeric. Take one portion daily.

3. Drink 2 ounces of aloe vera juice mixed with $\frac{1}{2}$ teaspoon of ground bay leaf twice daily.

4. Fill size 00 capsules (available at drugstores or health food stores) with turmeric. Take 2 capsules a few minutes before meals, 2–3 times daily, or put the same amount of turmeric in your food 2–3 times daily.

5. Herbal Formula—Mix 1 part guduchi, 1 part shardunika, 1 part kutki, and 2 parts punarnava. Take 1 teaspoon of the mixture 2–3 times daily with warm water. (You can purchase these herbs from the Ayurvedic Institute; phone number: 505-291-9698.)

Diet for Immune System Enhancement and Chronic Fatigue Syndrome

Milk Products—Active yogurt

Vegetables—**Garlic**, spinach, carrots, kale, sweet potatoes, pumpkin

Fish—Mackerel, salmon, herring, sardines

Spices—*Turmeric,* fenugreek, *ginger,* cumin, cinnamon

Teas (use separately or together)—**Chaparral (leaf), pau d'arco (inner bark)**, suma root, peach seed, *astragalus,* gentian, *dandelion,* licorice root, St. John's wort

Other—Shiitake/maitake/ling zhi (reishi) mushrooms, red wine, royal jelly, **aloe vera juice or gel**, grapefruit seed extract, spirulina, chlorella, flaxseed oil

Garlic Compound— Peel 30 cloves of garlic and let them rest 15 minutes before further handling. Place in a blender or food processor, add a small amount of water, and blend using short bursts until homogenized. Add 1 part homogenized garlic to 20 parts water; drink 2 glasses a day. Refrigerate garlic for further use.

Olive Leaf Compound—Squeeze the juice of a whole organic lemon. Place in a blender along with the lemon seeds and $\frac{1}{2}$ of the lemon rind. Add $1\frac{1}{2}$

cups of orange juice and 1 tablespoon of cold-pressed, extra-virgin organic olive oil. Blend ingredients at high speed for 2 minutes. Filter the mixture through a strainer to separate the juice from the pulp and discard the pulp. Divide the juice into three portions. Take 1 portion of juice (perhaps adding a little water) with 1 "Original Olive Leaf Extract" capsule (Ameriden; phone number: 888-405-3336) before breakfast, before lunch, and before dinner. Do this for 14 days, pause for one week, and then repeat again for 14 days. Continue this cycle until the chronic symptoms have abated. (Do not take if on allopathic antibiotics, prednisone, Zovirax, or amino acids.)

Avoid—Wheat and gluten, milk, corn

Osteoporosis Diet

Vegetables—Spinach, collards, turnip greens, beet greens, Swiss chard, celery, salad, carrots, cucumber (with peel)

Fruits—Apples, pears, grapes, dates, raisins, peaches, pineapple, figs

Legumes—Black beans, lima beans (pre-soak all beans overnight)

Fish—Pilchard, fresh sardines, herring, salmon, mackerel

Nuts—Almonds, peanuts, hazelnuts, cashews

Grains—Oatmeal, whole wheat, millet, buckwheat, alfalfa

Other—Honey (not heated in processing and from organic fields), ricotta cheese, Parmesan cheese, brick cheese, yogurt, chlorophyll/spirulina/chlorella supplement, hijiki/wakame/kelp seaweeds, tea made from horsetail and *Lobelia inflata* (steeped 10 minutes); wheat/barley grass

Avoid—Coffee, soft drinks, diuretics, excess red meat, sugar, excess salt, tomatoes, eggplant, bell peppers

⁘

Materia Medica

S pices are the greatest healers in the plant kingdom and we need to understand the tremendous contribution that these gifts of nature have made throughout the centuries in the science of health. In the United States, we tend to think that the primary role of spices is as additives to make food taste better. In traditional cultures, the foods have a complexity of tastes that is quite different from the food one is accustomed to eating in a typical American setting.

The art of preparing food in traditional cultures such as India, China, and the Middle East, just to mention three of the most familiar, does not focus on merely creating a great taste experience. It also ensures that the *energies* of the different foods used in a meal are all integrated and that the process of digestion is optimally stimulated and functioning properly. In addition, these traditions use spices as "daily herbal medicines" to strengthen the immune system, cleanse tissues, and integrate all functional systems. In this sense, every meal acts as a general stimulus for healing processes and serves to prevent future health issues by maintaining optimal health.

I became aware of this healing aspect of food while studying and working in Nepal in Ayurvedic and Tibetan clinics. I was amazed at the general standard of health in a country that has had severe economic problems for many years. There were virtually none of the chronic degenerative diseases that plague our society. The primary health issues stemmed mainly from the extreme poverty and working conditions that most people endured, including a laborious sixteen-hour work day, seven days a week, beginning at a very early age. It was obvious that for those people who could afford proper nourishment, diet played an important role in their health. In Nepal, the food is prepared traditionally, by hand, with prayerful intentions and long preparation times, allowing the right food combining and proper cooking. Many of the spices presented here are used daily.

Spices are used not only in cooking but also directly as medicinal substances, alone or as a part of herbal formulas. In the Middle Eastern traditions of medicine, prescriptions using spices as medicinal remedies far outweigh any other form of natural therapy.

The European tradition of using spices as medicine has a long history that has survived in what we call "folk medicine" and in traditional forms of naturopathic medicine still used in natural health care. The use of spices in Europe originated from two sources: the Crusades, when Europeans first encountered the use of Middle Eastern spices in daily cooking, and the impact of the Islamic and Greek medical sciences, which flourished in Spain during the medieval period. The Islamic and Greek traditions became refined into an extensive body of knowledge and an effective medical practice in the Christian monastic communities that served the surrounding populations. This tradition extended from Norway down through Christian Europe. Many monasteries served as hospitals and grew extensive herbal gardens, which produced medicinal substances. After the Reformation (in the sixteenth century) destroyed the majority of monasteries and almost four centuries of medical knowledge, the use of spices was relegated mostly to the kitchen.

Spices may come from different parts of the plant, such as the root, seed, bark, or leaf. The roots and seeds contain the greatest powers of transformation and life. One might say that root and seed processes dominate the life of the plant—the root as the plant's living foundation and the seed as the end product and fulfillment of the plant's life. The leaves, stem, and bark of a plant all have specialized medicinal properties, but ultimately serve the root and seed processes of the plant. The oil we use, such as olive oil, comes from the seed of the plant.

EASTERN AND MIDDLE EASTERN SPICES
Olive Oil

Olive oil is one of the great healers of the plant kingdom. Its healing effects have been recorded in all Classical medical traditions around the world for the last 3,000 years. Whether used in cooking or massaged into the skin, it helps the body build cells and restore worn-out tissues. Olive oil primarily supports the functions of the liver and improves digestion while relieving inflammation in the digestive system. It is used for diarrhea, colic, worms, food poisoning, and gas pains. Olive oil is not fattening, as many believe, because it helps the body to digest fats and fatty foods more completely.

Olive oil helps the bowels function normally and removes any congestion of the bile, which is produced in the liver. When the liver is sluggish or not functioning as well as it should, we can develop problems with cholesterol. Olive oil helps prevent heart disease caused by faulty liver functions, which can lead to cholesterol problems and hardening of the arteries. It has been proven to reduce "bad" cholesterol and increase "good" cholesterol as well as to soften gallstones.

Olive oil reduces excess heat in the body and soothes the nerve system. This is why it is so good for the skin and hair. Many cultures massage the skin and hair with olive oil to heal small wounds, give new life to the skin, nourish the hair and scalp, and help restore peace and balance to those suffering from nervous disorders.

Because the skin quickly absorbs olive oil and because this oil lowers heat and fights inflammation and infections, olive oil is used externally to reduce fevers and help heal measles, scarlet fever rashes, and burns. Olive oil also supports the kidney and bladder functions and helps with fluid retention. By supporting the liver and kidneys, it has been shown to be effective in lowering blood sugar in adult-onset diabetes.

Olive oil should be an essential part of your health program. It can be used for frying because its chemistry doesn't change when subjected to high temperatures. You can use it on salads or just take one teaspoon to one tablespoon of olive oil with meals, once or twice a day. An olive oil massage is very good for the general health of the skin and is used extensively in Eastern and Middle Eastern cultures for babies, young children, and women during and after pregnancy.

Garlic

Garlic has been a used as a health food as well as a powerful medicine in all Western and Eastern cultures for many centuries. It holds a central place in the Classical medical literature. Garlic is a powerful antimicrobial and is used to treat bacterial, viral, and yeast infections by enhancing the immune system. It contains elements that rejuvenate and build up all of the body's tissues and functions by reducing the factors that break down the health of the cells, including the effects of stress and nervousness. It is an excellent blood and tissue cleanser and works through the lymphatic system as an immune enhancer. Furthermore, it's helpful in cases of influenza, colds, bronchitis, ear infections, and pneumonia, due to its antibiotic effect and its ability to dispel phlegm.

Note, however, that it is not good to use garlic internally when there are any acute heat processes like fever in the case of colds and influenza. In conditions where fever is present, you can use it very successfully by crushing it into olive oil and applying it externally (see Colds and Flu in Part Two).

Garlic is very effective for improving digestion, eliminating parasites and intestinal yeast infections, stabilizing cholesterol, and reducing colic. Garlic promotes circulation and is used for support in heart problems involving arteriosclerosis, palpitation, and high blood pressure. It is used in rheumatoid arthritis and other connective tissue problems, including hemorrhoids and edema. Garlic is also a very good remedy for the reproductive organs in dealing with impotency. It increases all the metabolic processes and biological heat in the body, which is one of the reasons why it is so healthy.

Garlic, like many food-medicines, is good to use in the daily preparation of food as well as in medicinal preparations. By using these natural healers as part of daily nutrition, we help maintain a strong and healthy foundation.

Coriander

Two separate parts of the coriander plant are medicinal and both are used in the preparation of food and as a potent medicine. One is the fresh leaf, referred to as cilantro, and the other is the seed, which can be used whole in cooking and teas or can be ground into a powder for medicinal purposes. Coriander reduces the effects of heat and inflammation in the body. This is unusual because most spices raise biological heat in order to increase the digestive functions and stimulate tissues. Because of coriander's ability to neutralize excess heat, it is used for such ailments as allergies, hay fever, skin rashes, hives, burns, stomach irritation, and sore throat, as well as urinary tract problems like bladder infections.

When used in cooking, coriander increases digestion and the assimilation of food while at the same time reducing the natural heat in hot foods like chilis and tomatoes. Coriander can be used for diarrhea, vomiting, and heartburn. It works mainly through the blood and has a cleansing effect on bodily tissues as well as enhancing the immune system. It is one of the very "balanced" spices (like ginger, turmeric, cinnamon, fennel, and cardamom) that promote better integration of all body and mind functions.

Turmeric

Turmeric is a healing spice that works on all tissues of the body and cleanses the bioenergetic channels that connect one organ system to another. It strongly enhances the immune system and is an excellent natural antibiotic and antiviral substance, as well as an effective antitumor remedy. It cleanses the blood and lymphatic system, removes toxins, helps rid the body of parasites, and stimulates the building of new blood cells.

Turmeric is also an excellent digestive, aiding in the digestion of proteins and correcting all metabolic processes in the seven tissue systems (see Digestive Dysfunction in Part Two). Turmeric can be used for stomach ulcers, liver problems, high cholesterol, indigestion, poor circulation, skin disorders, and allergies.

Ginger

In Eastern medical traditions, ginger is called the "king of spices," due to its wonderful properties. It is the most harmonious of all spices and clears the bioenergetic channels that connect one organ system to another, as well as stimulating and supporting the metabolism of all seven tissue systems (see Digestive Dysfunction in Part Two). Ginger is very good for the digestion and for digestive issues such as constipation, diarrhea, anorexia, nausea, and vomiting. It's a heart tonic that cleanses the blood and helps remove blood clots. Ginger has a healing effect on respiratory system problems as well as on high fever and works well in skin diseases and in joint problems like arthritis.

Cinnamon

Cinnamon is a harmonizing, integrating, and strengthening spice. Like ginger, it could be considered an almost universal medicine. It supports weak constitutions and is a pain reliever as well as a heart, kidney, and circulatory stimulant. It helps clear all bioenergetic channels that connect one organ system to another and stimulates immune processes, especially in the mucous membranes where it works to expel phlegm and mucus from the body. Cinnamon is a very good digestive that not only promotes digestion but also supports all aspects of tissue metabolism. Cinnamon helps stabilize blood sugar and is often used by those who have low blood sugar issues or diabetes.

Cardamom

Cardamom is one of the best digestives and stimulates the primary digestive metabolism. It also stimulates the mind and enhances the power of concentration while promoting feelings of well-being and peacefulness. It is strongly integrating and harmonizing. Cardamom stimulates and stabilizes all the bioenergies that flow through the energetic channels and connect one organ system with another. It reduces the phlegm produced in the mucous membranes connected to digestive processes, and therefore is good for asthma. In addition, cardamom can be used for alleviating "nervous" digestion, improving poor nutrient absorption, and strengthening the Kidney System, and for treating colds, coughs, bronchitis, and asthma.

Black Pepper

Black pepper supports all primary biological functions. (Buddha recommended that his monks should start each morning by taking seven black peppercorns as a strengthening medicinal!) It helps balance the bioenergetics of the body by stimulating the energies of the Kidney System as well as being a powerful digestive stimulant that supports all metabolic processes. It also cleanses the intestinal tract of toxins and parasites, and clears congestion in the mucous membranes.

Black pepper counteracts "cold processes" in the organ and tissue systems and strengthens immunity. Taken with food, black pepper antidotes the cold energies of raw foods and salads as well as dairy products. It is used to treat problems in the mucous membranes, such as sinus congestion, bronchitis, tonsillitis, and colds. Furthermore, it strengthens weak digestion and stimulates the heart.

EUROPEAN SPICES AND HERBS

Oregano

Oregano was first used extensively in ancient Greek medicine. It strengthens and stimulates the immune system, especially the mucous membranes, and is often used in infections involving the mouth, gums, tonsils, lungs, and sinuses, where it helps to liquefy and expel mucus. Oregano is also used for skin conditions, such as fungus, sores, and skin ulcers, and as a compress for insect bites and stings. In traditional European medicine, oregano is used to treat rheumatism and joint issues like arthritis, due to its ability to reduce inflammation, relieve pain, and cleanse joints and muscles of toxins and poisons.

Oregano should not be taken during pregnancy as it is also used to help expel the afterbirth placenta and therefore is not appropriate until *after* the birth has taken place.

Sage

Sage has two main medicinal properties: it reduces excess secretions from the body's tissues, especially the mucous membranes and connective tissues, and it works on the mind and emotional states. Sage is very good for colds and flu, as it dries up mucus, and relieves all issues involving the lymphatic system, such as swollen lymph glands, laryngitis, and sore throats. In the connective tissues, it works to eliminate sores and skin ulcers and to stop bleeding. Sage also provides a calming and integrating effect on the mind and emotions by promoting clarity and "cleansing" the mind of old emotional blockages. In many Native American medical traditions, sage is used to cleanse negative influences and for spiritual purification.

Rosemary

Rosemary is one of the universal healers of the European spice family. Its wonderful properties extend from the mental and emotional realms to all physiological processes and the immune system. Rosemary is a strong heart and circulatory stimulant that helps stabilize heart functions and improve circulation, while it builds blood and helps resolve anemia. It strongly improves primary biological energy in the body's systems and restores brain, adrenal, and nerve system functions, as well as promotes calmness and well-being. In addition, rosemary helps resolve fatigue, stress from overwork, depression, anxiety, memory loss, and nervous disturbances. It works on the immune system through the mucous membranes and connective tissues and is used for whooping cough, colds, flu, bronchitis, and asthma, as well as for all infections, tissue repair, swollen lymph glands, wounds, sores, and burns. In the digestive sphere, rosemary helps with high cholesterol, strengthens the liver, works on gallstones, and helps resolve chronic enteritis (inflammation of the small intestine) and colitis (inflammation of the large intestine). Rosemary also supports the reproductive organs, helping to resolve conditions such as vaginal discharge, lack of menstruation, and painful menstruation.

Thyme

Thyme is another great general healer. It works strongly on the immune system through the kidney, adrenal, and lung systems, promoting biological strength in the body and resistance to all diseases through increased immunity. It is effective in the repair of tissues and in resolving all infections as a strong antibacterial, antifungal, and antiviral substance. For the upper respiratory tract, thyme is used to expel phlegm from the lungs, bronchial tubes, and sinuses and in the treatment of bronchitis, wheezing, allergic asthma, whooping cough, and sore throat. It works well on mental and emotional issues, such as depression, nervous exhaustion, obsessive thoughts, and the effects of stress, including lack of sexual desire. Thyme is also used to relieve the pain of neuralgias (nerve pain), rheumatism, and arthritis. It strongly supports the digestive processes and is used for building up the intestinal flora, which leads to a reduction of *Candida* yeast in the intestinal tract; and for treating colitis, enteritis, and slow digestion. Thyme works well on the skin in cases of psoriasis and dermatitis (skin infection) and supports the skin's connective tissues. It is also used for insect and animal bites. Lastly, thyme is a good reproductive organ stimulant and helps with abnormal vaginal discharge, lack of menstruation, and painful menstruation by stimulating and decongesting the uterus.

Fennel

Like rosemary and thyme, fennel is a universal healer. The whole plant can be used when boiled or baked, or it can be eaten raw in salads; the seeds are used as a spice. Fennel works primarily on the urogenital system by stimulating and harmonizing the functions of the reproduction organs, kidneys, and bladder. These systems are responsible for all basic immunity and for the strength of the immune system, as well as for basic cell nutrition and the body's primary biological energies. Fennel is used to reduce uric acid in the urinary system, which helps dissolve kidney and bladder stones, and supports urination. In the reproductive organs, fennel is used to help resolve conditions such as uterine congestion, lack of menstruation, problems with the breast tissues, estrogen insufficiency, and menstruation cramps. Fennel stimulates the stomach, spleen, and intestines, working well on digestive issues such as colic, nausea, vomiting, food poisoning, spasms and cramps in the intestines, and gas. The stomach has a direct connection with the mucous membranes of the lungs, so fennel is also used to expel phlegm and deal with asthma, bronchitis, and wheezing. Fennel strongly activates the immune system and connective tissues by cleansing the body of toxins and clearing parasites and is a good preventative for colds and flu.

Basil

Basil is another of the many plants that became known medicinally in the European Middle Ages through contact with the East and Middle East. In the Ayurvedic traditions of India, basil is considered to be a sacred plant. There, it is customary to grow basil inside the home as a way of blessing the house and all who dwell there. Science has validated the wisdom of growing basil in the home and has found that it releases ozone into the air and absorbs positive ions while energizing negative ions, just as advanced air purifiers do. Basil is a harmonizing herb that integrates both the body and mind and enhances all of the vital biological energies. It opens the heart to the spiritual aspects of consciousness and promotes awareness, love, and compassion. Basil is also a strong immune enhancer and strengthens fertility and the functions of the reproductive system. It energizes the senses, reduces stress in the nerve system, strengthens nerve tissue, and helps the memory. In addition, basil works effectively on digestive processes and reduces mucus in the respiratory tract, making it helpful in colds, flu, fever, sinus problems, and lung issues. Basil supports liver functions as well and helps them heal joint and muscular problems.

*Thank you for sharing this experience
with us. In the introduction to this
book, I told you how this book came
to be written—how it all began.
I can't tell you how it will end, for this
book is about life. Books about life
have no endings, only beginnings.
So let us begin again together—
today—each on our own book
of life and all beautiful things.*

—David

Bibliography

Medicine and Science

Anatomi og Fysiologi, Bind I og II. Copenhagen, Denmark: Nyt Nordisk Forlag, 1975.

Bohm, David. *Wholeness and the Implicate Order.* London: Routledge, 1995.

Briggs, John. *Fractals: The Patterns of Chaos.* New York: Simon and Schuster, 1992.

Capra, Fritjof. *The Tao of Physics.* London: Harper Collins, 1992.

Ganong, W. F. *Review of Medical Physiology.* Los Altos, CA: Lange Medical Publications, 1981.

Gatz, Arthur. *Manter's Essentials of Clinical Neuroanatomy and Neurophysiology.* Philadelphia: F. A. Davis, 1970.

Hamer, Ryke Geerd, Dr. med. *Kurzfassung der Neuen Medizin.* Koln: Amici di Dirk Verlagsgesellschaft, 1994.

Hauschka, Rudolf. *Ernahrungslehre: Zum Verstandnis der Physiologie der Verdauung und der Ponderablen und Imponderablen Qualitaten der Nahrungsstoffe.* Frankfurt am Main: Vittorio Klostermann, 1982.

Hoffmeyer, Jesper. *En Snegl paa Vejen, Betydnings Naturhistorie.* Copenhagen, Denmark: Omverden/Rosinante, 1993.

Kervran, Louis C. *Biological Transmutations.* New York: Swan House, 1972.

Konig, Karl. *Earth and Man.* Wyoming, RI: Biodynamic Literature, 1982.

Leviton, Richard. *The Physician: Medicine and the Unsuspected Battle for Human Freedom.* Charlottesville, VA: Hampton Roads, 2000.

Margulis, Lynn, and Doris Sagan. *Mikrokosmos, Fire Milliarder Aars Udvikling.* Copenhagen, Denmark: Munksgaard, 1990.

Mathiasen, Lund og Lunau. *Fysiologisk Atlas—En Studiehaandbog.* Copenhagen, Denmark: Medicinsk Forlag, 1975.

Meinig, George E. *Root Canal Cover-Up.* Ojai, CA: Bion Publishing, 1998.

Moore, Keith L., and T. V. N. Persaud. *The Developing Human: Clinically Oriented Embryology.* Philadelphia: WB Saunders, 1993.

Murphy, Christine, ed. *The Vaccination Dilemma.* New York: Lantern Books, 2002.

Rapp, Doris J. *Is This Your Child's World?* New York: Bantam Books, 1996.

Richards, W. Guyon. *The Chain of Life.* Essex, England: CW Daniel, 1954.

Roy, Ravi, and Carola Lage-Roy. *Homeopatisk Behandling af Vaccinationsskader.* Copenhagen, Denmark: Klitrose, 1992.

Schmidt, Paul. *Krebs: Eine Vollblockade im Zellerneuerungs-Zentrum des Gehirns.* Germany: Bonn & Fries, 1983.

Smith, Emil L., Robert Hill, Robert Lehman, Robert Lefkowitz, Philip Handler, and Abraham White. *Principles of Biochemistry.* New York: McGraw Hill, 1983.

Thompson, Richard. *Foundations of Physiological Psychology.* New York: Academic Press, 1967.

Food and Herbal Therapy

Bonder, Nilton. *The Kabbalah of Food.* Boston: Shambhala Publications, 1998.

Culpeper's Complete Herbal. Hertfordshire, England: Wordsworth Editions, 1995.

Gallavardin, Jean-Pierre. *Repertory of Psychic Medicines with Materia Medica.* New Delhi: World Homeopathic Links, 1983.

Harper-Shove, F. *Prescriber and Clinical Repertory of Medicinal Herbs.* Devon, England: Health Science Press, 1952.

Holmes, Peter. *The Energetics of Western Herbs: Integrating Western and Oriental Herbal Medicine Traditions,* 2 vols. Boulder, CO: Artemis, 1989.

Hutchens, Alma R. *A Handbook of Native American Herbs.* London: Shambhala, 1992.

Junius, Manfred M. *Practical Handbook of Plant Alchemy: How to Prepare Medicinal Essences, Tinctures and Elixirs.* New York: Inner Traditions, 1985.

Lu, Henry C. *Chinese System of Food Cures: Prevention and Remedies.* New York: Sterling Publishing, 1986.

Messegue, Maurice. *Mine Laege Planter.* Copenhagen, Denmark: Borgen, 1975.

Morningstar, Amadea, and Urmilla Desai. *The Ayurvedic Cookbook.* Santa Fe, NM: Lotus Press, 1991.

Pedersen, Mark. *Nutritional Herbology.* Bountiful, UT: Pedersen Publishing, 1991.

Pitchford, Paul. *Healing with Whole Foods: Oriental Traditions and Modern Nutrition.* Berkeley, CA: North Atlantic Books, 1993.

Vogel, A. *The Nature Doctor.* Bodensee, Germany: Verlagsanstalt Merk & Co., 1960.

Wood, Matthew. *The Book of Herbal Wisdom: Using Plants as Medicine.* Berkeley, CA: North Atlantic Books, 1997.

Psychology and Spirituality

Avalon, Arthur. *Shakti and Shakta.* New York: Dover Publications, 1951.

Guenther, Herbert V., and Leslie S. Kawamura. *Mind in Buddhist Psychology.* Emeryville, CA: Dharma Publishing, 1975.

Hozeski, Bruce. *Hildegard of Bingen's Scivias.* Santa Fe, NM: Bear & Company, 1986.

Kalupahana, David J. *The Principles of Buddhist Psychology.* Albany, NY: State University of New York Press, 1987.

Kaplan, Aryeh. *The Bahir.* London: Jason Aronson, 1995.

Kaplan, Aryeh. *Sefer Yetzirah: The Book of Creation.* York Beach, ME: Samuel Weiser, 1997.

King, Richard. *Early Advaita Vedanta and Buddhism.* Albany, NY: State University of New York Press, 1995.

Kochumuttom, Thomas A. *A Buddhist Doctrine of Experience.* New Delhi: Motilal Banarsidass Publishers, 1989.

Kuvalayananda, Swami. *Pranayama.* Philadelphia: The Sky Foundation, 1978.

O'Murchu, Diarmuid. *Quantum Theology: Spiritual Implications of the New Physics.* New York: Crossroads Publishing, 1999.

Prokes, Mary Timothy. *Toward a Theology of the Body.* Grand Rapids, MI: William B. Eerdmans, 1996.

Rajagopalachari, C. *Mahabharata.* Bombay: Bharatiya Vidya Bhavan, 1990.

Rama, Swami, Rudolph Ballentine, M.D., and Swami Ajaya. *Yoga and Psychotherapy: The Evolution of Consciousness.* Glenview, IL: Himalayan International Institute, 1976.

Sardello, Robert. *Facing the World with Soul: The Reimagination of Modern Life.* Hudson, NY: Lindisfarne Press, 1992.

Sardello, Robert. *Freeing the Soul From Fear.* New York: Riverhead Books, 1999.

Tulka, Tarthang. *Reflections of Mind.* Emeryville, CA: Dharma Publishing, 1975.

Whitmont, Edward C. *Psyche and Substance: Essays on Homeopathy in the Light of Jungian Psychology.* Berkeley, CA: North Atlantic Books, 1980.

Classical and Traditional Medicine

Semitic

Carmy, Shalom (ed.). *Jewish Perspectives on the Experience of Suffering.* Jerusalem: Jason Aronson, 1999.

Chishti, Hakim G. M. *The Traditional Healer: A Comprehensive Guide to the Principles and Practice of Unani Herbal Medicine.* Rochester, VT: Healing Arts Press, 1988.

Moinuddin, Abu Abdullah Ghulam. *The Book of Sufi Healing.* New York: Inner Traditions, 1985.

Rosner, Fred. *Medical Encyclopedia of Moses Maimonides.* Jerusalem: Jason Aronson, 1998.

Rosner, Fred. *Encyclopedia of Medicine in the Bible and Talmud.* Jerusalem: Jason Aronson, 2000.

Weintraub, Simkha Y., ed. *Healing of Soul, Healing of Body: Spiritual Leaders Unfold the Strength & Solace in Psalms.* Woodstock, VT: Jewish Lights Publishing, 1994.

Ayurveda

Dash, Bhagwan. *Alchemy and Metallic Medicines in Ayurveda*. New Delhi: Concept Publishing, 1986.

Dash, Bhagwan, and Lalitesh Kashyap. *Basic Principles of Ayurveda*. New Delhi: Concept Publishing, 1989.

Dash, Bhagwan. *Concept of Agni in Ayurveda*. Varanasi: Chowkhamba: Sanskrit Series Office, 1971.

Dash, Bhagwan. *Materia Medica of Indo-Tibetan Medicine*. New Delhi: Classics India Publication, 1987.

Dash, Bhagwan. *Ayurveda for Mother and Child*. New Delhi: Delhi Diary Publishers, 1988.

Dwarakanatha, C. *Introduction to Kayachikitsa*. Veranasi: Chaukhambha Orientalia, 1986.

Kumar, Abhimanyu. *Child Health Care in Ayurveda*. New Delhi: Sri Satguru Publications, 1999.

Lad, Vasant. *Ayurveda: The Science of Self-Healing*. Albuquerque, NM: Lotus Press, 1984.

Sharma, S. N. Valdya. *Concept of Jatharagni in Ayurveda*. Jaipur: Publication Scheme, 1992.

Chinese Medicine

Beinfield, Harriet, LAc, and Effrem Korngold, LAc, OMD *Between Heaven and Earth: A Guide to Chinese Medicine*. New York: Ballantine Books, 1991.

Hammer, Leon. *Dragon Rises, Red Bird Flies: Psychology & Chinese Medicine*. New York: Station Hill Press, 1990.

Kaptchuk, Ted J., OMD *The Web That Has No Weaver: Understanding Chinese Medicine*. Chicago: Congdon & Weed, 1983.

Larre, Claude, Jean Schatz, and Elisabeth Rochat de la Vallée. *Survey of Traditional Chinese Medicine*. Columbia, MD: Traditional Acupuncture Foundation, 1986.

Mann, Felix. *Acupuncture: The Ancient Chinese Art of Healing*. London: William Heinemann, 1974.

Porkert, Manfred. *The Theoretical Foundations of Chinese Medicine: Systems of Correspondence*. Cambridge, MA: The MIT Press, 1985.

Seem, Mark, with Joan Kaplan. *Bodymind Energetics: Toward a Dynamic Model of Health*. Rochester, VT: Healing Arts Press, 1989.

Yu, Lu K'uan. *Taoist Yoga*. York Beach, ME: Samuel Weiser, 1973.

Tibetan

Donden, Dr. Yeshi. *Health through Balance: An Introduction to Tibetan Medicine*. New York: Snow Lion Publications, 1986.

Dummer, Tom. *Tibetan Medicine and Other Holistic Health-Care Systems.* New York: Routledge, 1988.

Khangkar, Lobsang Dolma. *Lectures on Tibetan Medicine.* New Delhi: Library of Tibetan Works and Archives, 1986.

Spiegelman, Marvin and Mokusen Miyuki. *Buddhism and Jungian Psychology.* Phoenix, AZ: Falcon Press, 1987.

Anthroposophical

Husemann, Friedrich, and Otto Wolff. *The Anthroposophical Approach to Medicine,* Vol. 1 and 2. Hudson, NY: The Anthroposophic Press, 1982.

Steiner, Rudolph. *The Healing Process: Spirit, Nature and Our Bodies.* Hudson, NY: The Anthroposophic Press, 2000.

Steiner, Rudolf, and Ita Wegman. *Extending Practical Medicine.* London: Rudolf Steiner Press, 2000.

Von Heydebrand, Caroline. *Childhood: A Study of the Growing Child.* Hudson, NY: The Anthroposophic Press, 1995.

Western Classic/Traditional

Dodt, Colleen. *Natural Babycare: Pure and Soothing Techniques for Mothers and Babies.* Pownal, VT: Storey Books, 1997.

Hildegard, Saint (translated by Priscilla Throop). *Hildegard von Bingen's Physica.* Rochester, VT: Healing Arts Press, 1998.

Kaiser, Josef. *Das Grosse. Kneipp Hausbuch.* Munchen, Germany: Knaur, 1975.

Marquardt, Hanne. *Reflekszonearbejde paa Foden.* Heidelberg, Germany: Thaning & Appel, 1975.

Russell, David. *The Names of Life: The Practice of Being in Classical Medicine.* Doctoral Thesis, Madison University, 2002.

Schulz, Hugo, and Ferd Sauerbach. *Ursachen und Behandlung der Krankheiten.* Heidelberg, Germany: Karl F. Haug Verlag, 1983.

Strehlow, Wighard, and Gottfried Hertzka. *Hildegard of Bingen's Medicine.* Santa Fe, NM: Bear & Company, 1987.

Wiese Sneyd, Lynn. *Holistic Parenting: Raising Children to a New Physical, Emotional, and Spiritual Well-Being.* Los Angeles: Keats Publishing, 2000.

Index

About the Authors

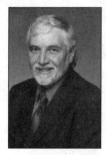

David Russell, M.F.A., Ph.D., has been teaching Classical Medical disciplines and spiritual psychology in Europe, Nepal, and the United States, as well as diagnostics and homeopathy in naturopathic schools in Denmark and Norway, for the past thirty years. He has worked for the Chaplains ministry at the Tucson Medical Center, at the Wilmot Federal Prison in Tucson, and has his own practice in Denmark and Tucson, Arizona.

Dr. Russell has studied and practiced with Classical masters in Europe, Nepal, and the Middle East. He holds certifications in reflexology, homeopathy, acupuncture, Islamic medicine, Ayurvedic medicine, biochemistry, iridology, and Kneipp therapy. He received training in the Netherlands in the field of anthroposophical medicine as a therapeutic teacher *(heilpedagog)* and homeopath working with multi-handicapped children. He is also qualified in Chinese and Tibetan medicine.

Dr. Russell is a founding member of the Danish Society for Integrated Medicine and was instrumental in establishing the three major clinics for Integrated Medicine in Denmark. He has worked for the Royal Danish College of Agriculture in Copenhagen on research in agricultural homeopathy, and has taught in several nurse-training programs in Denmark. He has been an affiliate faculty member of the Interfaith Theological Seminary, and a faculty member of the Arizona School of Acupuncture and Oriental Medicine. He is a medical consultant for Stop-Unge, a Danish clinic for drug and alcohol abuse.

He lectures for the International Congress of Probiotic Medicine, the American Academy of Biological Dentistry, the Cancer Congress, and on spirituality and medicine at the University of Arizona. He has chaired a seminar series at Barnes & Noble on holistic medicine.

Dr. Russell is also the founder and director of the non-profit organization CARITAS TRADITIONALIS—an international project (NGO) whose goal is to create self-sustainable medical presence in economically depressed communities. You can visit Dr. David Russel at his website www.davidnrussell.com.

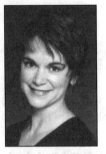

Lynn Wiese Sneyd is the author of *Holistic Parenting: Raising Children to a New Physical, Emotional and Spiritual Well-Being* and coauthor of *How Happy Families Happen: Six Steps to Bringing Emotional and Spiritual Health into Your Home.* Her articles, essays, and poetry have appeared in various newspapers and magazines around the country. Currently, she directs the Author Promotions division of the Russell Public Affairs Group. A graduate of the University of Wisconsin-Madison, Lynn resides in Tucson, Arizona, with her husband and two daughters.